"Preparing for the arrival of a new baby can seem a nearly monumental task, especially for working parents trying to balance the roller-coaster ride of pregnancy or the adoption process along with dual careers and all of life's routine responsibilities. High expectations and little guidance can make the first trip to a baby superstore an overwhelming and emotional experience for even the most successful among us. With *Baby Lists*, Elaine Farber helps expectant mothers and fathers cut through the clutter and cut to the chase with an invaluable resource to help prepare house and home for the joyful arrival of their most valuable new addition."

—Linda Mason, founder and chairman of
Bright Horizons Family Solutions and
author of *The Working Mother's Guide to Life*

BABY LISTS

BABY LISTS

What to Do and What to Get to Prepare for Baby

Elaine Farber

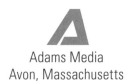

Adams Media
Avon, Massachusetts

Published by Adams Media, an F+W Publications Company
57 Littlefield Street
Avon, MA 02322
www.adamsmedia.com

ISBN-10: 1-59869-238-0
ISBN-13: 978-1-59869-238-9

Printed in the United States of America.

J   I   H   G   F   E   D   C   B   A

Library of Congress Cataloging-in-Publication Data
Farber, Elaine
Baby lists / Elaine Farber.
p.   cm.
ISBN-13: 978-1-59869-238-9 (pbk.)
ISBN-10: 1-59869-238-0 (pbk.)
1. Infants—Care. 2. Parent and infant. 3. Infants—Development.
4. Child rearing. I. Title.
HQ774.F33 2007
649'.1220284—dc22
2007002029

This publication is designed to provide accurate and authoritative information with regard to the subject matter covered. It is sold with the understanding that the publisher is not engaged in rendering legal, accounting, or other professional advice. If legal advice or other expert assistance is required, the services of a competent professional person should be sought.
—From a *Declaration of Principles* jointly adopted by a Committee of the American Bar Association and a Committee of Publishers and Associations

Many of the designations used by manufacturers and sellers to distinguish their product are claimed as trademarks. Where those designations appear in this book and Adams Media was aware of a trademark claim, the designations have been printed with initial capital letters.

This book is available at quantity discounts for bulk purchases.
For information, please call 1-800-289-0963.

*I want to dedicate this book to my husband Alan,
my two boys, David and Marc,
and my daughter, Carrie.
You all mean so very much to me.
You are the loves of my life.*

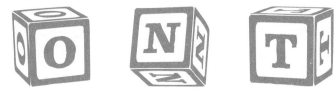

Part 3. Books, Videos, DVDs, and Music

ACKNOWLEDGMENTS

First, thanks to my husband Alan for his dedication through all the hours he spent researching the book-writing process, writing proposals, and contacting publishers. The book took a long time to complete, and I understand his frustration with my procrastination. I'm grateful to him for putting up with me through the process.

I want to thank my daughter, Carrie, who also loves to write, for pushing me when I became complacent about finishing the book, and for all her helpful suggestions as I wrote it.

My gratitude goes to my mother for the financial backing she has given to put the book together. Without her help, the book would not have materialized.

This book would never have been finished without my editor, Sharon Hamm, who has been such a big help. I am grateful for her patience and understanding, for all of her help with how to work my computer, for some of the writing she aided with, and much more. It's been a pleasure to work with her.

I'd also like to acknowledge all my clients, some of whom have become very good friends, for the privilege of caring for their newborns and creating the opportunity for me to become familiar with all of the baby products on the market today. I want to mention two people in particular: Donna Downing, a former client, who encouraged and inspired me to write this book in the first place; and Dena Fischer, another former client, who has been there to answer my questions and guide me through this whole process.

And I would like to thank Dr. Allan Levy, a very special man, who gave me the confidence I needed to pursue this endeavor. He has always been there to answer my questions and steer me in the right direction.

My appreciation to you all!

Elaine Farber

It was 1968 when my husband and I brought our first baby home from the hospital. I held her in the car. Infant seats weren't invented yet. When we got home, we put her in the middle of our bed and stood on each side so she wouldn't roll off. We looked at each other and said, "Now what do we do?!"

I was very young and clueless. In those days, Dr. Spock's book, *Baby and Child Care*, was the bible to new parents. It took awhile but I eventually calmed down. Looking back, it is amazing that she managed to survive. I'm surprised she didn't melt because of all the layers of clothes I put on her. I wanted her to have the best of everything and purchased many things I would never need or use.

Twenty-eight years later, I stood in a hospital room with tears in my eyes as I looked at my first grandson. Our son-in-law turned to us and said, "This is a life-altering moment for all of us—we have just become parents and you have become grandparents." It was really fun to watch them as they sterilized everything and made everyone wash their hands before they could hold the baby. When her third baby was just a few weeks old, she said, "Can anyone take him? I have to pick up Max at soccer."

One of the most amazing aspects of becoming a grandparent was to see the change in what is available for babies. Shopping for the first grandchild was a real learning experience. There was so much more out there—so many choices and so many decisions. How could we possibly know what was a necessity and what was hype and advertising? My tendency was to buy everything, which is, of course, not very practical.

Reading *Baby Lists: What to Do and What to Get to Prepare for Baby* made me wish that this book had been available for all of us. Elaine Farber has done an amazing job of compiling everything you ever wanted or needed to know about preparing for a new baby. *Baby Lists* covers absolutely every aspect of becoming a new parent. The important issues of pregnancy, birth, health, safety, and security are covered extensively. The book is so comprehensive it even mentions hangers for their darling little outfits.

When another daughter had twins, we were thrust into a new and different experience—not the least of which was buying two of everything. The little girls were so tiny—it would have been so helpful to read this book's section on "preemie pacifiers." (Who knew?) Elaine Farber is thorough. She provides explanations of every baby necessity and luxury. She gives realistic descriptions of items as well as specific brands and Web sites. For first-time parents (and grandparents) it's a lot to comprehend all at once. Don't be overwhelmed by the amount of information contained in the book. Use it as a reference and guide. Relax and enjoy your baby, knowing that when a question arises, you have the encyclopedia of baby paraphernalia at your fingertips.

Melinda Kanter-Levy
Founder of Marin Day Schools

Preparing for a baby can be overwhelming and expensive. With so many things to think about, such as what products you'll need and how to choose a pediatrician, you can be at a loss for answers to the questions you have. Within this book, you'll find many of those answers.

Baby Lists offers real-world information and shopping lists to help you through this important time. As an all-in-one resource, this book is unique. It is the only book of its kind that consists primarily of lists—lists presented in a format that is easy to read and navigate through. This complete guide of checklists offers information about everything you will need to do and shop for as you prepare for your baby's arrival. The content is detailed and comprehensive yet concise and accessible—no more going through endless paragraphs and chapters to find the information you are looking for. With the help of *Baby Lists*, your baby can come home to a safe, complete, and calm environment.

Part 1, "Becoming-Baby-Ready Lists," helps you make choices about important aspects of baby's life before and immediately following birth, and continuing through the first months and years. This section includes important tools of all sorts—tools to help you choose a hospital and put together your birth plan, select a pediatrician, pack for the hospital, assemble a complete first-aid kit for your home and nursery, and even buy and pack the diaper bag. This section also includes a chapter all about childproofing your home so your baby is safe from the minute she arrives, and complete questionnaires and forms to help you select a nanny.

Part 2, "Necessities and Nice-Things-to-Have Lists," is a trustworthy resource to help you choose merchandise from cribs and car seats to books and bouncy seats. With this handy reference guide, you can identify and locate products that are necessary, as well as those that are just nice to have. For example, Chapter 11, "Newborn Necessities," tells you what you need in your nursery, right down to how many of each item to purchase. The lists also include the name of the top recommended products, their manufacturers, and Web sites where you can find the product, so you can research before you buy. And if you can't find a product at its listed Web site, simply go to *www.google.com* or *www.froogle.com,* type the name of the product and the manufacturer into the site's search option, and the product Web site should pop right up on your screen. You also will find a summary list of key Web sites for baby items in the Appendix at the end of the book.

Part 3, "Books, Videos, DVDs, and Music," offers you a comprehensive list of resources to choose from as you build your library of books and music to entertain, soothe, and educate your baby and growing child.

You'll want to keep the book close by as you begin to plan for your new baby. And be sure to have it handy to refer to when you're deciding what, and how much, to buy. Happy parenting!

Part 1

Becoming-Baby-Ready Lists

Chapter 1

Choosing a Hospital

Depending on where you live and where your doctor has privileges, you may have the option of deciding between several hospitals, or only one hospital might be available to you. In either situation, be sure to check out the hospital well in advance of your due date. If you become familiar with the hospital and its protocol, you will feel more comfortable when it comes time for you to deliver your baby.

FACTORS TO CONSIDER

Location

Consider location when you are choosing a hospital. Ideally, you want the best hospital that is closest to your home. Before you go into labor, map out the most direct route to the hospital you select. If you live in an area where there might be a problem taking the direct route, plan an alternate route as well. Also, make sure the hospital you choose is covered under your insurance plan.

Getting to the Hospital

If you should go into labor and cannot reach your partner, or you are alone when you go into labor, you'll need a plan for getting to the hospital. Have a relative or friend standing by who can take you to the hospital on short notice. Keep this person's phone number with you, as well as directions to the hospital, wherever you go: You can't predict where or when you're going to go into labor!

Obstetrician and Pediatrician Privileges

Make sure your obstetrician has admitting privileges at the hospital of your choice (not all doctors can practice at every hospital in your area). Also find out whether the pediatrician you've selected has privileges at the hospital. If your pediatrician does not have privi-

leges there, find out whether there will be a pediatrician on staff who will take care of your baby until you're discharged.

Level-Three Nursery

If you are having a high-risk pregnancy or are pregnant with multiples, choose a hospital with a level-three nursery. Only a level-three nursery is equipped to put a baby with respiratory problems on a ventilator. This procedure is called intubation. If the hospital where you deliver doesn't have a level-three nursery and your baby has complications after birth, the baby will have to be transferred to another hospital that's equipped to handle such emergencies.

GETTING TO KNOW THE HOSPITAL

Familiarize yourself with the hospital early in your pregnancy. By visiting well before you go into labor, you'll find out the hospital's policies on delivery, birthing rooms, visitors, siblings, and nursery status; for example, when visitors are allowed, what different types of birthing rooms are available, and whether your older child can come to visit. Having this information will ensure that you'll get the kind of birthing environment you want. Most hospitals offer a tour of the obstetrical floor, and you can ask these questions when you have your tour. Call the hospital and arrange to take a tour of the postpartum unit, the nursery, and the delivery area. Tours are usually given once or twice a month in the evenings. If you've taken a tour of the units, the hospital will seem more familiar to you when you arrive in labor.

You'll also have to preregister with the hospital a month in advance of your due date. If you are expecting multiples, it's a good idea to preregister two months in advance of your due date. Registration forms are available from your doctor or directly from the hospital.

1. What is the patient-to-staff ratio? Does one nurse care for both Mom and baby? What is the maximum number of patients each nurse has per shift?

   _____

   _____

2. What levels of staffing are used on the postpartum floor and in the nursery? Are all the nurses RNs? How are LVNs (licensed vocational nurses) and nursing assistants used in the nursery and on the postpartum floor?

   _____

   _____

3. What type of security system does the hospital use to ensure my safety and the safety of my baby? Are video cameras or sensor bands used? What type of identification should all hospital personnel be wearing?

   _____

   _____

4. How many people, besides my partner, are allowed to be present during labor and delivery? (Some expectant moms want their other children, parents, sister, or best friend present during labor and delivery. This question makes sure the hospital will allow for that.)

   _____

   _____

5. Are there birthing rooms? Do I remain in the same room throughout my hospital stay (labor, delivery, and postdelivery)?

   _____

   _____

6. If I do not remain in a birthing room, what other types of rooms are available? Are all the rooms private, or are some semiprivate? What are the costs per day for a private or semiprivate room?

   _____

   _____

Taking a tour of the hospital before delivering my baby was so worth it. I knew just where to go and what to expect when I arrived in labor.—Jennifer

7. What type of bed is used during delivery? Is a breakaway bed available? (The breakaway bed allows you to deliver in the sitting-up position.) Outside of having a C-section, under what circumstances would I deliver in an operating room?

_____

_____

8. Is there always an anesthesiologist at the hospital, or is one on call?

_____

_____

9. Are walking epidurals given? (If you don't know the definition of a walking epidural, ask your medical professional to explain.)

_____

_____

10. Are showers or baths with my partner allowed during labor?

_____

_____

11. Is a neonatalogist or pediatrician on staff in the hospital at all times?

_____

_____

12. Is the nursery prepared to handle level-three emergencies, or would the baby be transferred to another hospital? Which hospital receives transfers?

_____

_____

13. How will my pediatrician know I've delivered my baby?

_____

_____

14. What is the hospital's rooming-in policy? Is it possible to send the baby to the nursery any time during the day or night so that I can get some rest? If the baby remains with me throughout the night, does the hospital require another adult to be present?

_____

_____

15. Does the hospital have in-house lactation consultants available? How often will the lactation consultant visit?

_____

_____

16. What are visiting hours? Are there restrictions on visitors? Are siblings allowed to visit at any time? Are siblings allowed to spend the night? Do visitors have to scrub and gown before entering the room when the baby is present?

_____

_____

17. Am I allowed to bring in my own electrical appliances (hair dryer, radio, shaver, etc.)?

_____

_____

18. Are there any instructional videos available for viewing after I deliver? (Many hospitals have videos on breastfeeding, giving baby a bath, characteristics of the newborn, and so on. Viewing the videos and becoming familiar with these subjects will help answer some questions that may come up after you get home.)

_____

_____

QUESTIONS TO ASK WHEN YOU PREREGISTER

1. What is the parking situation? Does the hospital have parking validation for Dad and visitors?

_____

_____

2. When I come to the hospital in labor, do I stop at admitting or go directly to the maternity floor? (If you are already preregistered, usually you can go right to the obstetrical floor.)

_____

_____

3. Many hospitals lock the front door after 11 p.m. and require you to enter through the emergency room entrance. If I arrive at the hospital after 11 p.m., which entrance do I go through?

_____

_____

4. Are the telephones accessible twenty-four hours a day? What are the hours for incoming calls? Can I make outgoing calls at any time?

_____

_____

5. What classes does the hospital offer regarding exercise, childbirth, child care, and breastfeeding? When are the classes given, where do you pre-register, and what are the fees? Do I need my doctor's permission to attend any of these classes? (For some exercise classes, you'll need written permission from your doctor before you can attend.)

_____

_____

Knowing what to ask while taking my hospital tour provided me with answers to all of my pertinent questions.—Sandra

WHAT TO DO WHEN YOU ARRIVE AT THE HOSPITAL IN LABOR

If you are already preregistered when you arrive at the hospital, follow the instructions you have been given. Usually this means going directly to the maternity floor. If you haven't preregistered, you may be required to stop by the admitting office. If you are in heavy labor, however, even if you haven't preregistered, go directly to the maternity floor. You can do the admitting paperwork later.

When you arrive on the maternity floor, check in with the nurse at the desk. The nurse will help you and your husband with any necessary maternity paperwork. The nurse will then take you to a labor-and-delivery suite or birthing room, orient you to your surroundings, and introduce you to your labor-and-delivery nurse.

Chapter 2
Creating a Birth Plan

M any expectant moms want to have a say in their care during pregnancy, labor, and delivery. A birth plan is a simple, non-confrontational way for you to make your care preferences clear to everyone involved. Many medical professionals welcome your input. It shows that you are taking an active role in your pregnancy and the birth of your baby. Every hospital and every health-care professional has a certain protocol to follow, so if you don't have a birth plan, you'll receive standard treatment.

It is important to remember that even though you have a birth plan, and you have discussed your preferences with your health-care professionals, unexpected circumstances or emergency situations can arise during labor and delivery. Your birth plan will never over-ride medically necessary procedures. You should always have the utmost confidence that your doctors are doing what's best for you and your baby. However, don't be afraid to ask your doctors questions if you don't understand what they are doing or saying.

Although there are many choices to make and things to consider, birth plans are best kept short and to the point. Only include things on your final birth plan that are very important to you. For instance, do you want anesthesia during the birth? How long do you want to stay in the hospital?

Following is a guide to creating your own birth plan. Once you have your plan the way you want it, make sure you go over it with your doctor or health-care professional at your next visit.

Remember that a birth plan is a statement of preference, not a binding contract. If at any time you change your mind about something that's stated in your birth plan, your wishes should be respected.

HOW TO SET UP A BIRTH PLAN

1. Choose a Title
   Sample title: "Birth Plan: My Preferences During Labor, Delivery, and My Hospital Stay"

2. Set Up the First Page
   - First, middle, and last name
   - Name of primary health-care provider
   - Name of hospital/center where you plan to deliver
   - Due date
   - Coach (e.g., partner, friend)
   - Other support

3. Write a Letter of Introduction
   Include the date and a salutation for your doctor or healthcare professional.

   ### Sample letter
   Dear Dr. (name of doctor) and the staff of (hospital name):
   I look forward to sharing the birth of my baby with you. I have created the following birth plan to help you understand my preferences during my labor and delivery. I understand that there may be circumstances that will not allow my birth plan to be followed; however, assuming all goes as planned, these are my preferences. If you have any questions or suggestions, please let me know.
   Sincerely,
   (your name)

4. Indicate Specific Preferences
   Use the following lists as a reference, and check off your preferences. If you wish, you can type up your own birth plan to indicate only your choices.

Having a birth plan really helped me convey to my doctor and nurses what my preferences would be during labor and delivery.—Melinda

ENVIRONMENT

○ I would like to give birth in a birthing room.
○ I would like to give birth at home.
○ I would like to bring my own music to play during labor.
○ I would like the environment to be kept as quiet as possible.
○ I would like the lights to be kept low during my labor and delivery.
○ I would like to have a VCR available.

DESIGNATED OBSERVERS

I would like the following people with me during labor and delivery

○ Partner (coach)   ○ Doula   ○ Friends   ○ Children   ○ Relatives

ENEMAS

○ I would like to have an enema upon arriving at labor and delivery.
○ I would prefer to avoid an enema, and the shaving of pubic hair. (These procedures are no longer standard at many hospitals.)

LABOR—FIRST STAGE

○ I expect doctors and hospital staff to discuss all procedures with me before they are performed.
○ If I go past my estimated due date, I would prefer not to have labor induced unless it is necessary for me or the baby.
○ I prefer not to be separated from my partner (coach) at any time during labor and delivery.
○ I prefer to wear my own nightgown during labor and delivery.
○ I would like to be free to walk around during labor.
○ I would like to have ice chips and fluids by mouth during the first stage of labor.
○ I prefer to keep the number of vaginal exams to a minimum.

○ I would like to take a bath or shower with my partner (coach) during labor.

○ I wish to labor freely in the birthing tub or shower.

○ I would prefer no students or residents to be present during labor and delivery.

LABOR INDUCTION/AUGMENTATION

○ As long as the baby and I are not in any distress, I would like to be free of time limits and avoid induction unless it is medically necessary.

○ Do not rupture my membranes artificially unless it turns out to be medically necessary.

○ If labor is not progressing, I would like to have the amniotic membrane ruptured before other methods, such as Pitocin, are used to augment labor.

○ If induction or augmentation is necessary, I would like to try the following:

❑ Prostaglandin gel   ❑ Pitocin

❑ Castor oil   ❑ Breast stimulation

❑ Enema   ❑ Sexual intercourse

❑ Walking   ❑ Stripping or breaking membranes

MONITORING

○ I do not wish to have continuous fetal monitoring unless it is medically necessary for the baby.

○ I would like the baby to be monitored externally.

○ I would like the baby to be monitored intermittently using a Doppler.

○ I would like the baby to be monitored intermittently using a fetoscope.

ANESTHESIA/PAIN MEDICATION

○ Please do not offer pain medication; I will request it, if needed.

○ I would like to avoid all narcotics, if possible.

○ Before considering an epidural, and if the situation warrants, I would like to try an injection of narcotic pain relief (Nubain, Demerol, Stadol, or a similar medication).

○ I prefer an epidural to narcotic pain medication.

○ I would like to have an epidural as soon as permissible.

○ I would like to have a light-dose (walking) epidural.

○ I would like the epidural to wear off slightly as I approach full dilation and the pushing stage.

○ I would like to try one or more of the following for pain management:

- ❑ Acupressure
- ❑ Relaxation
- ❑ Breathing techniques/distraction
- ❑ Hot/cold therapy
- ❑ Hypnosis
- ❑ Massage
- ❑ Bath/shower

LABOR—SECOND STAGE: DELIVERY

○ I would like to choose the position in which I give birth.

○ I do not want to use stirrups while pushing.

○ I would like my partner (coach), nurses, or both to support me and my legs as necessary during the pushing stage.

○ I would like to deliver in a birthing pool, and I have made arrangements to rent one for the birth.

○ As long as the baby and I are fine, I would like to push at my own pace.

○ I would like a mirror so I can see the baby's head when it crowns.

○ I would like to touch the baby's head when it crowns.

○ In the event of an assisted birth, I would prefer the use of forceps rather than vacuum extraction.

○ In the event of an assisted birth, I would prefer vacuum extraction rather than the use of forceps.

EPISIOTOMY

○ I would prefer not to have an episiotomy unless it is absolutely required for the baby's safety.

○ I would appreciate guidance on when to push and when to stop pushing, so the perineum can stretch to avoid tearing.

○ I would prefer an episiotomy rather than a tear.

○ I would rather risk a tear than have an episiotomy.

○ I would like perineal massage to avoid tearing.

○ Please suture tears only if necessary.

○ I would like a local anesthetic to repair a tear or an episiotomy.

BIRTHING EQUIPMENT

I would like to have the following birthing equipment available to me during labor:

- ○ Birthing bed
- ○ Squatting bar
- ○ Birthing stool
- ○ Birthing pool/tub
- ○ Birthing chair

CESAREAN SECTION

- ○ Unless absolutely necessary, I would like to avoid a Cesarean delivery.
- ○ If a Cesarean delivery is indicated, I would like to be fully informed and participate in the decision-making process.
- ○ I would like my partner (coach) present at all times if the baby requires a Cesarean delivery.
- ○ I wish to have a spinal/epidural for anesthesia so I can be conscious during the delivery.
- ○ I wish to have general anesthesia for a Cesarean delivery.
- ○ If it is possible, please do not strap my arms to the table during the procedure.
- ○ I would like to have one hand free to touch the baby.
- ○ If possible, I would like to breastfeed the baby immediately after birth.
- ○ I want my partner (coach) to be able to record the birth.
- ○ If the baby is not in distress, I would like him/her to be given to me (or my coach) immediately after birth.

POSTBIRTH

- ○ I would like the baby placed on my stomach or chest immediately after birth.
- ○ I prefer that the umbilical cord stop pulsating before it is cut.
- ○ My partner (coach) would like to cut the cord.
- ○ I would like (other) to cut the cord.
- ○ I prefer not to have routine Pitocin after the birth.
- ○ Please show me the placenta after it is delivered.
- ○ I would like to hold the baby while I deliver the placenta and any tissue repairs are made.
- ○ I would like to breastfeed the baby immediately.
- ○ After the birth, I prefer to be given a few moments of privacy to urinate on my own before being catheterized.
- ○ I would like to donate the umbilical cord blood, if possible.
- ○ I would like to bank the umbilical cord blood, and I have made arrangements to do so.

NEWBORN CARE

- ○ I would like to hold the baby for a least fifteen minutes before he or she is examined, photographed, and so on.
- ○ I would like to have the baby evaluated and bathed in my presence.

- If the baby must be taken from me to receive medical treatment, my partner (coach) or some other person I designate will accompany the baby at all times.

POSTPARTUM CARE

- I would like a private room, if possible.
- I would like my partner (coach) or a person I designate to spend the night with me.
- Unless required for health reasons, I would like to have the baby room-in with me at all times.
- I would like the baby with me during the day and in the nursery at night unless otherwise specified.
- I would like my baby brought to me for feedings only.
- I would prefer the baby be kept in the nursery and brought to me upon request.
- I would like my other children to have free visitation access.
- I would like my hospital stay to be as long as possible.
- I would like my hospital stay to be as short as possible.
- I would like to have access to my chart and the baby's chart.

BREASTFEEDING

- I plan to breastfeed and would like to begin nursing shortly after birth.
- I would like to see a lactation consultant about breastfeeding.
- I would like to breastfeed on demand.
- Unless it's medically necessary, I do not wish to have any bottles given to the baby (including glucose water or plain water).
- I do not plan to breastfeed the baby.

FORMULA FEEDING

- I plan to formula feed my baby.
- Use any formula the pediatrician recommends.
- I would like a specific formula given to my baby.
- I would like my baby fed on demand.
- I would like my baby fed on a schedule.
- Glucose or plain water may be given to my baby.
- I don't want the baby to have glucose or plain water.
- A pacifier may be given to my baby.
- I don't want the baby to have a pacifier.

CIRCUMCISION

○   I do not want the baby circumcised.

○   I would like the baby to be circumcised before we check out.

PHOTO/VIDEO

○   I would like to take still photographs during labor and the birth.

○   I would like to make a video recording of labor, the birth, or both.

I felt very comfortable knowing I had a say in the care and feeding of my baby.—Angie

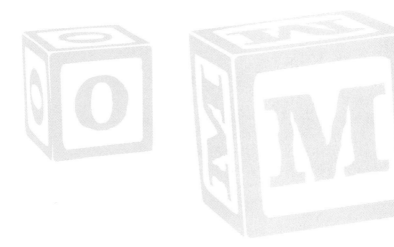

Chapter 3

Finding and Interviewing a Pediatrician

Choosing the right pediatrician is one of the most important decisions you make for your child. In your baby's first year, you will visit your pediatrician approximately six times for well-baby check-ups, and five times for other reasons such as illness or injury. Do you want a pediatrician who offers choices and allows you to decide which option works best for you? Or would you be more comfortable with a doctor who has strong opinions and gives a lot of direction? You want to find a pediatrician in a practice that makes you feel confident and comfortable. Your pediatrician should also be warm, compassionate, and open to your thoughts and feelings, and you should share similar views on child rearing. Choose the right pediatrician, and he might be able to treat your child from birth through adolescence.

HOW TO BEGIN YOUR SEARCH

It's a good idea to begin your search for the right pediatrician during your sixth month of pregnancy. Making your final decision during your seventh or eighth month will make things much easier for you when the baby is born. If you are looking for a pediatrician for the first time, are not happy with your present pediatrician, or are moving and have to find a new pediatrician, here are suggestions to follow:

1. Compile a list of candidates by asking friends, relatives, coworkers, neighbors, and your obstetrician for recommendations. Ask them whether their pediatrician really seems to enjoy working with their children.

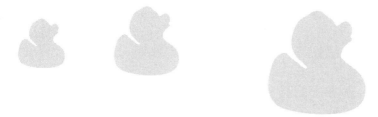

2. Call the medical schools located in your area and ask to speak to the chief resident in pediatrics. Ask whom she would take her child to.

3. Get names from your obstetrician's office of doctors who are certified by the American Board of Pediatrics, local medical society, hospital referral service, or the national office of the American Academy of Pediatrics.

4. Send a request for information with a self-addressed, stamped envelope to the Pediatrician Referral Department, AAP, P.O. Box 927, Elk Grove Village, IL 60009-0972. Be sure to tell them which region of the state or country you're interested in.

If you know the sex of your child, you might want to consider choosing a pediatrician of the same gender. When children become teenagers, they often feel more comfortable with a doctor of the same sex. Another thing to think about is the age of the doctor. If you choose an older doctor, ask whether retirement is in the near future and, if so, who will take over the practice.

1. How does your child respond to your pediatrician? Is your child happy or fearful when the doctor comes in the room?

   _____

2. Does your doctor seem to know about the latest medical techniques? Was there ever an occasion when you needed advice about a particular problem? Were you satisfied with your doctor's answers? Did your pediatrician have to confer with another source?

   _____

3. Does your doctor welcome questions? Does he take the time to answer the questions thoroughly? Do your appointments ever seem rushed?

   _____

4. Does your pediatrician take time to discuss problems and listen to your concerns? Is he interested in discussing topics other than physical problems, such as your child's emotional and psychological health?

   _____

5. Is the office staff patient and helpful? Is there an advice nurse available to answer questions? Does the staff or doctor return phone calls promptly?

   _____

WHAT TO DO AFTER YOU HAVE YOUR RECOMMENDATIONS

Different doctors have different approaches to child rearing, so interview several pediatricians. You want to make sure you select the one that best suits your family's needs. Call to make appointments to interview the pediatricians you're considering. Arrange to meet pediatricians individually and in person during the final months of your pregnancy. If possible, both parents should attend the first meeting. Don't interview pediatricians over the phone. Only a face-to-face meeting will let you know whether a pediatrician has the type of personality and philosophy about child rearing that you are seeking. If the pediatrician doesn't have the time to talk to you in person, he probably won't have the time during an office visit to answer your questions. That's not the kind of doctor you're looking for. It is very important to feel comfortable with the pediatrician you choose. Keep in mind that some pediatricians will charge for a consultation.

In addition to talking with the pediatrician, you'll want to ask the doctor's staff some questions. When you make your appointment, be sure to ask whether there will be a staff member available to answer questions.

When you are deciding on a pediatrician, make sure the office is conveniently located. Imagine driving across town, through heavy traffic, with a sick and miserable child.

Never feel afraid or embarrassed to ask questions of a potential pediatrician. Remember, your child is your most precious gift.

1. How long have you been in practice?

2. Are you a member of the American Academy of Pediatrics or any other specialty organization?

3. Where did you go to school?

4. What do you like best about your job?

5. Do you have any subspecialties?

6. Do you belong to a group practice? If so, how many doctors are there in the group?

7. What are your office hours?

8. What are your days off?

9. How can I reach you in an emergency?

10. If you can't be reached in an emergency, what procedure should I follow?

11. Who covers for you if you're not available?

12. What hospitals are you affiliated with?

13. After I give birth, will you or someone from your practice be visiting the baby in the hospital?

14. Is there an after-hours clinic and, if so, when is it open?

15. Do you encourage parents to call for routine/nonemergency questions?

16. Will you be available for discussions on my child's behavioral development—tantrums, discipline issues, social development, and so on?

17. What are your feelings regarding the following topics:

Breastfeeding

Bottle feeding

Starting solid foods

Weaning baby from breast or bottle

Circumcision

Getting baby to sleep

Vitamins

Antibiotics

Alternative medicine

Preventative medicine

Immunizations

Taking baby out in public

Traveling with baby

Daycare in private homes or centers

18. What child-care books do you recommend?

1. How does the office handle phone inquiries?

2. Is there a specific time for parents to call with questions, or is there an open advice line during office hours?

3. Is there a twenty-four-hour answering service that will connect to a doctor?

4. Does the staff dispense its own advice or relay the doctor's comments?

5. How far in advance do I have to schedule appointments?

6. If my child is sick, can I get an appointment that same day?

7. Are any diagnostic procedures performed on-site, such as blood work or x-rays?

8. If the lab is not on-site, what lab do you recommend?

9. How soon after birth is the first well-baby visit?

10. How often are well-baby visits?

11. Do newborns and well children have to wait in the same waiting room with sick children?

12. After we arrive for an appointment, what is the typical waiting time before we see the doctor?

13. What happens if I miss a scheduled visit? Can I easily reschedule?

14. Does the office mail out reminders for scheduled immunizations and checkups?

FEES AND METHODS OF PAYMENT

1. Do you have a list of fees for the various services that are provided?

   _____

2. Are immunization shots extra, or included in the office visit charge?

   _____

3. What insurance coverage does your office accept?

   _____

4. How are billing, laboratory charges, and insurance claims handled?

   _____

5. Do you accept checks or credit cards?

   _____

Knowing I could rely on the pediatric staff made me feel very comfortable about the pediatric office I chose to take care of my baby.—Melissa

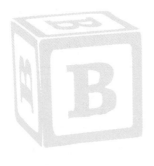
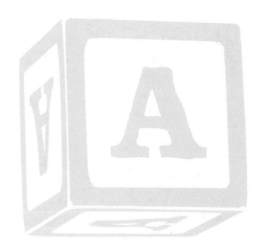

THINGS TO ASK YOURSELF AFTER THE INTERVIEW

1. Do you and this pediatrician share similar views on topics such as breast-feeding, circumcision, working mothers, daycare, and so on? If not, is the pediatrician open to different opinions or other approaches?

2. Does the pediatrician seem to be up-to-date on the latest medical advances?

3. Did you feel comfortable with the doctor?

4. Did the doctor welcome questions and take the time to address your concerns?

5. Did the pediatrician and office staff treat you courteously or curtly?

6. Is the office conveniently located?

7. Is there ample parking?

8. How long were you kept waiting?

9. Did the waiting room and the examination room have toys and books?

10. Was everything clean?

11. How helpful were the nurses and support staff at the office?

After you decide on a pediatrician, call the office and let them know your approximate due date. If you know in advance that you are going to have a C-section, and your chosen pediatrician has privileges at the hospital where you are going to deliver, he or one of his partners should be in attendance.

Chapter 4
Packing for the Hospital

P acking for the hospital or birth center is fun and exciting, but you don't want to leave anything behind! To give yourself plenty of time, it's best to begin packing your birth bag by your thirty-fourth week. Pack one bag for labor, and another for postpartum and baby. Keep handy—perhaps attached to the refrigerator door—a list of last-minute items to add to your bag just before you leave for the hospital. This way, you can be assured that even if you go into labor early, you will have everything you need to make yourself comfortable. The hospital might provide you with certain items, but they will charge you for almost everything, so you might wish to bring some of the necessities with you. If your partner plans to keep you company during your hospital stay, they should pack a small bag as well.

Not everyone will want or need all of the items on the lists; select the items you feel will be most helpful to you during your hospital stay. Check off the items as you pack them in your bags.

WHAT TO PACK IN YOUR LABOR AND DELIVERY BAG

○ Copies of Pre-registration Paperwork
   Keeping the paperwork with you will save time when you arrive at the hospital.

○ Birth Plan
   A birth plan details your preferences during labor and delivery, and after the baby is born (see Chapter 2).

○ Bathrobe
   A robe will come in handy if you want to go for a walk during early labor and after the baby is born. Don't bring your best robe because it might become soiled.

○ Slippers
  The hospital will require you to have something on your feet when you are out of bed. Your own slippers will be more comfortable than the paper slippers the hospital gives you. Slip-on, nonskid slippers are the easiest to get into. You won't want to bend over to put on shoes or ballerina-type slippers after delivery, especially if you have a C-section.

○ Socks
  During labor, your feet might get cold. It's nice to have a pair of socks to warm them up.

○ Bathing Suit
  If your water hasn't broken, you can take a soothing bath or shower with your partner, and they can give you a massage to help with pain management.

○ Pillow
  Having your own pillow can be very comforting.

○ Hair Bands, Scrunchies, or Bobby Pins
  If you have long hair, you will want something to hold it away from your face.

○ Lip moisturizer or ChapStick
  Your lips can get very dry during labor, especially if you are given certain medications. Lip moisturizer or ChapStick will keep them moist and prevent them from cracking.

○ Massage lotions or oils
  Some women enjoy a massage during labor. Massage lotions or oils help you to relax.

○ Breath Mints or Lollipops

It's refreshing to have some breath mints or lollipops to suck on during labor because your mouth might get dry. Lollipops are better than hard candy, which can be a choking hazard.

○ Instant Coffee or Tea

It's easier and faster to get a cup of hot water than to purchase coffee or tea. This may come in handy especially for your partner or coach during a late-night delivery.

○ Snacks

You may be allowed to eat light snacks in the early stages of labor. Your partner or labor coach might also get hungry. Depending on the time of day, the coffee shop or cafeteria may be closed, so it's wise to pack a few munchies. Ask your doctor what type of snacks you can have during the early stages of labor.

○ Change for Vending Machines

Vending machines may be the only source of food in the hospital.

○ Watch with a Second Hand

Labor and hospital rooms usually have a large wall clock to time contractions, but you might want to bring your own watch with a second hand.

○ Eyeglasses

Bring regular glasses and reading glasses if you need them. Even if you wear contact lenses, you'll probably need or want to take them out at some point during your hospital stay.

○ Relaxation Materials

❑ Books/magazines ❑ Deck of cards

❑ Soothing-sounds machine ❑ MP3 player

❑ Games ❑ CD player and CDs

○ Tennis Ball or Rolling Pin

Some labor coaches recommend that you use a tennis ball or rolling pin for back massage during labor.

○ Birthing Ball

Leaning or sitting on a birthing ball can decrease the discomfort of contractions, relieve the pain of back labor, and aid the baby's descent into the birth canal.

○ An Object to Focus on During Labor

A picture of something or someone you love, or an object that is meaningful to you, can help keep your mind focused.

○ A Good-Luck Charm

Anything you feel brings you good luck can help mentally comfort you.

- Cameras and Accessories
  - Camera and film or memory card
  - Extra batteries or battery charger
  - Tripod

- Keys
  In this flurry of activity, don't lock yourself out of the house!
- Cell Phone and Charger
  You may want to alert family and friends that you are on the way to the hospital. Having your cell phone handy will make it easier for people to find you any time day or night.
- Plastic Bag
  If you feel nauseated, a plastic bag could come in handy in the car.
- Towels
  If your water breaks, the towels will protect the upholstery in your car.

On the way to the hospital my water broke. Thank goodness for the towels I brought along in the car to protect the seat.—Darla

- Packed Bags
  After spending all that time and energy packing your bags, you don't want to leave them at home.

PACKING FOR POSTPARTUM CARE

Having everything you need for postpartum care is just as important as preparing for your labor and delivery. You want to be as comfortable as possible after labor, so make sure you have the following items packed so that you can spend more time enjoying your new baby and less time worrying about the little details.

CLOTHING

- Two Nursing Gowns
  Hospital gowns tie in the back and make breastfeeding difficult. Wearing a nursing nightgown will make breastfeeding more comfortable and enjoyable. You'll want to have at least two gowns with you so that if one gets stained, you'll have a fresh one to change into.

○ Nursing Bras
Beginning right after delivery, wear nursing bras day and night for support and to help prevent stretch marks.

○ Panties
Bring comfy, loose-fitting panties. These are especially important if you end up having a C-section. Don't bring new, fancy panties. Even though you will be wearing sanitary pads, your panties will probably get stained.

○ Going-Home Outfit
Plan to wear loose, comfortable clothing for the ride home. Bring something that is easy to get into. Maternity clothes might be the most comfortable.
   ❑ Pants
   ❑ Top
   ❑ Socks or stockings
   ❑ Flat shoes
   ❑ Sweater or coat

Bringing along my own toiletries in travel-size containers gave me all the comforts of home. —Sally

TOILETRIES

Purchasing travel-size toiletries will save space in your bags. Also, it's nice to bring your own soaps, shampoos, and toothpaste so you'll enjoy your favorite brands, scents, and flavors.

○ Toothbrush and Toothpaste
○ Mouthwash
○ Soap or Shower Gel
○ Shower Puff
○ Shower Cap
○ Shampoo and Conditioner
○ Comb and Hairbrush
○ Deodorant
○ Body Lotion
○ Baby Powder for Mom to Freshen Up
○ Razor and Shaving Gel (you'll probably be able to see your legs again!)
○ Makeup and Hand Mirror
○ Emery Board

○ Nursing Pads

Nursing pads protect your bra and clothing from breast-milk leakage.

○ Lanolin Nipple Cream

Start using this right away to help prevent sore, cracking nipples.

○ Sanitary Pads

Bring hospital-sized sanitary pads with an adhesive strip that holds the pad to your panties. If you have a C-section, wearing a sanitary belt can be very uncomfortable. If you have a vaginal delivery, you will probably be in the hospital for two days and should bring about twelve pads. If you're having a planned C-section, you will probably stay for four days and should bring about twenty-four pads.

○ Tucks Pads

Tucks pads are used to relieve the pain of hemorrhoids, which are fairly common after giving birth.

○ Hot-Water Bottle

If you have an episiotomy, you may want to apply heat to the affected area. Some hospitals have heat lamps, but it often takes hospital staff a while to get the lamp to you, and the position you have to sit in is very uncomfortable.

○ Ice Bag

Some women prefer to apply ice to the area affected by their episiotomy. The hospital will charge you for disposable ice bags, so it's better to bring your own.

○ Personal Appliances

If you'd like to bring your hair dryer, curling iron, or hot rollers, or take along a fan to keep you cool, check beforehand whether the hospital will allow you to plug in electrical appliances.

○ Earplugs

If your baby goes back to the nursery at night, you might like having a pair of earplugs handy. It's hard to sleep, hearing all the usual hospital noises going on throughout the night.

○ Safety Pins

Invariably there will be something to pin up or pin closed.

○ Contact Lenses and Solution

If you wear disposable lenses, bring extra pairs.

○ Medications

If you are taking medications for a preexisting medical condition, bring them along and give them to the nurse. Otherwise, new prescriptions will be ordered at hospital prices.

○ Small Bedside Clock
Most hospital rooms have wall clocks, but it's nice to have a clock right by your bed that you can see easily, especially if you're breastfeeding.

○ Nursing Pillow
If you bring your nursing pillow, the lactation consultant can show you how to use it while you're sitting in bed or in a chair. She'll demonstrate the many different ways to position your baby on the pillow to achieve maximum nursing efficiency.

○ Phone Card
You might want to make some long-distance calls and charge them to your phone card.

○ Insurance Card
Notify your insurance company within twenty-four hours after your baby is born.

○ Address Book with Phone Numbers
You'll want to call many people after the baby is born. Be sure to record the number of your lactation consultant, pediatrician, and baby nurse or nanny, if you plan to use one.

○ Notepad and Pen
Write down questions you may have for the doctor or nurses regarding yourself or your baby. If the phone rings and you're busy, someone else can write down a message for you. Keeping track of visitors, flowers, and gifts can be very helpful when it comes time to write those thank-you notes.

○ Birth Announcements and Stamps
Some new moms like to get those birth announcements out right away!

○ Breastfeeding Book
Even though you probably read up on breastfeeding while you were pregnant, it's nice to have a reference close by after delivery.

○ Baby-Naming Book
Some parents don't have names picked out—even after nine months!

○ Baby Book
Record baby's footprints. Some moms like to record the events of labor, delivery, and their hospital stay while they are still fresh in their minds. If guests come to visit, they can sign the baby book.

○ Dried Fruit
Dried fruit, such as prunes or apricots, can help relieve postpartum constipation.

I'm so glad I brought some dried fruit along. It really helped relieve my constipation after delivery.—Anne

○ Extra Duffle Bag

Having an extra empty duffle bag will come in handy if you should receive gifts at the hospital.

○ Champagne

Even a nursing mother can have a glass of champagne to celebrate the birth of her baby.

○ Gift for Nurses

They always like a good box of candy. Having worked in two hospital maternity units, I'd suggest buying a one-pound box for each shift.

PACKING FOR PARTNER OR COACH

More and more frequently, partners or coaches are staying with Mom after the baby is born. To make their stay more comfortable, they should pack a little bag for themselves, which should contain the following items.

○ Change of Clothes

- ❏ Underwear
- ❏ Sweater or long-sleeved shirt
- ❏ Pajamas
- ❏ Robe
- ❏ Slippers
- ❏ Bathing suit: As mentioned previously, if Mom labors in the shower or tub, the partner or coach can jump in with her and give her a massage or rub her back to help with pain management.

○ Toiletries

- ❏ Toothbrush and toothpaste
- ❏ Deodorant
- ❏ Razor and shaving cream
- ❏ Aftershave

○ Other Necessities

- ❏ Wallet
- ❏ Change
- ❏ Watch
- ❏ Snacks
- ❏ Pillowcase for dirty clothes
- ❏ Medications: Hospitals won't dispense any medications to expectant or new fathers, partners, or coaches. You may wish to bring along Tylenol for tension headaches.

PACKING FOR SIBLINGS

If you have a child who's still in diapers, don't forget:

- ☐ Diapers
- ☐ Wipes
- ☐ Pull-ups

- ○ Change of Clothes
  Children will get dirty. A change of clothes can come in handy.

- ○ Pajamas
  Siblings who stay overnight at the hospital will be comfortable in their own PJs.

- ○ Favorite Blanket and Pillow
  Your child will sleep better with his or her own blanket and pillow.

- ○ Favorite Bedtime Story
  A favorite story can be very comforting to your child when she is sleeping in a strange place.

- ○ Stuffed Animal
  Many children can't go to sleep without their favorite stuffed animal.

- ○ Favorite Toys, Crayons and Paper, and Games
  Sitting around in a hospital room can get pretty boring. Having some familiar toys to play with will help keep your child occupied.

- ○ Favorite Video or DVD
  Some hospitals have VCRs or DVD players available.

- ○ Snacks and Juice
  Hungry kids are cranky kids. There may not always be food around, so have a few snacks handy.

- ○ Big Brother or Sister T-Shirt
  Siblings are very proud to show off their big brother or sister T-shirt.

- ○ Present for Sibling from Baby
  Getting a present from the new baby will not only help make your older child feel included in the celebration but also will help establish a bond between your older child and the new baby.

PACKING FOR BABY

- ○ Formula, Bottles, and Nipples
  If you don't want to feed your baby a ready-to-use formula or the brands the hospital has on hand, be sure to bring along a can of powdered formula. Powdered formula is the most like breast milk and digests easily. And there are no open cans of leftover formula to refrigerate! If you plan to use powdered formula, bring a few 4- or 8-ounce bottles with the nipples of your choice (see Chapter 21 for information about bottles). Ask the nurse for some bottles of

sterile water, and pour the desired amount into one of your own bottles. Add the right amount of powdered formula (one scoop to every 2 ounces of water unless otherwise specified by your pediatrician), and shake well to mix.

○ Vaseline

Vaseline will protect baby's bottom and also make it easier to wipe off baby's bowel movements. Meconium, baby's first bowel movement, is a sticky, tar-like substance that's very messy and hard to get off baby's bottom. Simply apply a thin layer of Vaseline after each diaper change, and the meconium will wipe off easily.

○ Diaper Wipes

The hospital will give you gauze pads that have to be moistened with water to wipe baby's bottom. Bring along some diaper wipes if you don't want to be bothered with getting up to wet the gauze pads each time you change a diaper.

○ Nail Scissors

Some babies are born with very long fingernails, but hospital nurses are not allowed to cut them, so you might want to do it before you go home. Doing this prevents baby from scratching his face. Also, babies like to suck on their fingers and hands to comfort themselves. If the nails are cut, you can leave the baby's hands uncovered.

○ Mittens

If you don't want to cut your baby's fingernails until you get home, you can cover your baby's hands with mittens.

○ Car Seat

Have the car seat properly installed before you go to the hospital. Read all instructions carefully; if you have any questions, your local police or fire station can demonstrate proper installation. When you leave the hospital, you will be required to sit in a wheelchair, and your baby will be placed in your arms. Installing the car seat beforehand will save time; just buckle baby in, and you're on your way.

Taking the time to have our car seat professionally installed before bringing our baby home from the hospital gave us great peace of mind.—Sue

○ Head and Body Support for Car Seat
Most car seats today come with a built-in head-and-body support system. (If your car seat doesn't, you should definitely buy one of these systems.) If your baby's head is not supported as you're driving, it will flop from side to side or down onto his chest. If this happens, baby's airway can become blocked, causing breathing difficulties. And if you turn sharply or stop suddenly, damage could be caused to the baby's head, neck, or spinal column. You can thread today's supports right into the car seat's safety-belt system. Here are two good support systems and where you can find them online:

● Boppy Nogan Nest Head Support by Boppy
Manufacturer Web site: *www.boppy.com*
● Total Body Support Set by Infantino
Manufacturer Web site: *www.infantino.com*

○ Extra Receiving Blankets
If your baby is small, or you don't have a body-support system in the car seat, tuck rolled-up receiving blankets on each side of the baby in the car seat.

My baby was small, and having extra receiving blankets to prop him up in the car kept his head from rolling down onto his chest.—Nancy

○ Going-Home Outfit for Baby
❑ Romper with feet or special going-home outfit. It's a good idea to bring two outfits in case one gets dirty before you leave the hospital.
❑ Booties
❑ Hat
❑ Receiving blanket
❑ Snowsuit if the weather is cold
❑ Outer blanket
❑ Small container of diaper wipes

(The hospital will supply diapers, so you don't need them.)

WHAT NOT TO BRING TO THE HOSPITAL

Just as it's important to take everything you need with you when you go to the hospital, it's equally important to leave other things at home. Leave the following items at home when you go to the hospital—they'll be much safer at home, and you'll have more peace of mind and be better able to focus on the important matters at hand.

1. Jewelry
   During the excitement of labor and delivery, jewelry can get lost or stolen. If you want to keep your engagement and wedding rings on, make sure they fit snugly. If they are loose, wear a ring guard or tape them to your finger.

2. Cash
   Except for some change for the vending machines, you really won't need any money.

3. Credit Cards
   Everything is charged to your hospital bill, so you won't need credit cards.

4. Work
   Leave laptops at home.

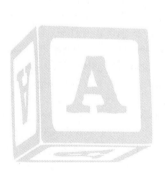
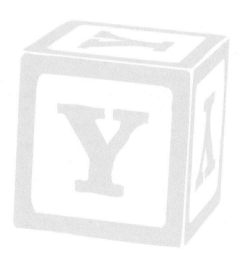

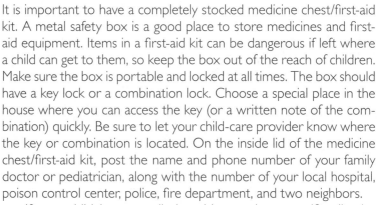

Chapter 5
Stocking Your Medicine Chest/First-Aid Kit

It is important to have a completely stocked medicine chest/first-aid kit. A metal safety box is a good place to store medicines and first-aid equipment. Items in a first-aid kit can be dangerous if left where a child can get to them, so keep the box out of the reach of children. Make sure the box is portable and locked at all times. The box should have a key lock or a combination lock. Choose a special place in the house where you can access the key (or a written note of the combination) quickly. Be sure to let your child-care provider know where the key or combination is located. On the inside lid of the medicine chest/first-aid kit, post the name and phone number of your family doctor or pediatrician, along with the number of your local hospital, poison control center, police, fire department, and two neighbors.

If your child has a medical problem such as specific allergies or some other life-threatening condition, always carry his medication with you and keep another prescription in your first-aid kit. If your child takes medicine regularly, or if he is sick and needs medication and a caregiver has to administer it, be sure the time, dosage, and method of administering the medication is written down and thoroughly explained. Have your caregiver keep a record of any medications given while you are at home or away. That way, you'll know what medications your child received, and the time they were administered.

Before you give your child any medication, unless the medication has been recently prescribed, always check with your pediatrician. The dosage will vary depending on your child's age and weight. These medications include over-the-counter medicines such as Tylenol, decongestants, antihistamines, cough syrups, and suppositories. Be sure to check the expiration date on medications in your first-aid kit frequently. Replace them as needed.

The following products should be in your medicine chest/first-aid kit. You can find all the products on this list online, or at your local pharmacy or grocery store. If you prefer to shop online, specific Web sites are provided for purchasing most of these products. Examples of specific brands of each product are bulleted.

With a fully stocked medicine and first-aid kit, I know I'm ready for almost any emergency that may arise.—Denise

MEDICINES, REHYDRATION FLUIDS, AND POISON ANTIDOTES

❍ Fever Reducer
A fever reducer is used to relieve pain and reduce fever caused by teething, illness, or immunization reactions.
- Infant Tylenol
  Vendor Web sites: *www.drugstore.com*; *www.walgreens.com*

❍ Decongestant
Decongestants help dry up stuffy, runny noses.
- To be prescribed by your pediatrician

❍ Antihistamine
An antihistamine can relieve itching and swelling from bug bites or allergic reactions.
- To be prescribed by your pediatrician

○ Cough Suppressant
A cough suppressant can help calm a persistent, nagging cough.
- To be prescribed by your pediatrician
○ Saline Eye Drops
Saline eye drops are used to wash foreign bodies out of the eye.
- Hypo Tears Lubricant Eye Drops
Vendor Web sites: *www.longs.com*; *www.walgreens.com*
○ Pedialyte Rehydration Fluids
Pedialyte rehydration fluids are used to treat dehydration caused by vomiting and infant diarrhea. Pedialyte Oral Electrolyte Maintenance Solution comes in liquid form for babies and popsicle form for older children.
- Pedialyte Oral Electrolyte Maintenance Solution
Vendor Web sites: *www.longs.com*; *www.walgreens.com*

When your child is sick and can't keep anything down or has diarrhea, Pedialyte rehydration fluids are the best. They replenish the electrolytes lost when your child is sick.—Maureen

○ Syrup of Ipecac
Syrup of Ipecac induces vomiting in cases of accidental poison ingestion. Always call your pediatrician or poison control center before you administer syrup of Ipecac. Syrup of Ipecac should only be administered under the supervision of a physician. In some cases, when the poison ingested is caustic, you do not want to induce vomiting.
- To be prescribed by your pediatrician
○ Activated Charcoal
Activated charcoal is used in cases of accidental poisoning when you do not want to induce vomiting. Activated charcoal helps to neutralize poisons. Always check with your pediatrician and poison control center before you administer this.
- To be prescribed by your pediatrician

LOTIONS, OINTMENTS, AND SOAPS

○ Mild Soap
Babies have sensitive skin. Keep a mild soap in the first-aid kit to wash off the many cuts and scrapes your child will encounter as she grows up.
- Baby Soap Bar by Johnson's Baby
Manufacturer Web site: *www.johnsonsbaby.com*

○ Antibacterial Ointments
Treat cuts or scrapes with antibacterial ointment, which reduces the possibility of infection.

- Neosporin First-Aid Antibiotic Ointment
- Polysporin First-Aid Antibiotic Ointment
  Vendor Web sites: *www.drugstore.com*; *www.longs.com*

○ Topical Calamine Lotion or Hydrocortisone Cream (1 percent)
These creams are used for insect bites and itchy rashes.

- Anti-Itch & Rash 1% Hydrocortizone Cream Plus Aloe by Rite Aid
  Vendor Web site: *www.drugstore.com*
- Calamine Lotion
  Vendor Web site: *www.drugstore.com*; *www.walgreens.com*

○ Hydrogen Peroxide
Clean cuts and scrapes with hydrogen peroxide to decrease the chance of infection.

- Hydrogen Peroxide Solution by Rite Aid
  Vendor Web sites: *www.drugstore.com*; *www.walgreens.com*

○ Rubbing Alcohol
Use rubbing alcohol for cleaning thermometers, tweezers, and other instruments.

- Isopropyl Rubbing Alcohol 70% by Rite Aid
  Vendor Web sites: *www.drugstore.com*; *www.walgreens.com*

○ Child-Safe Insect Repellent
Keep bugs and insects from biting your baby by applying an insect repellent.

- Baby Bug Block by Little Forest
  Vendor Web sites: *www.babyproofingplus.com*; *www.ourgreenhouse.com*
  Baby Bug Block uses an effective blend of ingredients that wards off insects without the use of chemical agents that may be harmful to baby's skin. With Little Forest your baby will enjoy safe, natural, and effective protection against insect bites.
- Citronella Bug Blend Bug Repellent Lotion by California Baby
  Manufacturer Web site: *www.californiababy.com*
  This nontoxic, DEET free, nonchemical, hypoallergenic formula repels bugs while it soothes existing bites and hydrates the skin.

OTHER NECESSITIES FOR FIRST-AID KIT

○ Calibrated Medicine Dispenser
A medicine dispenser is used for measuring and administering the proper dose of medications.

- Medicine Dropper by Safety 1st
  Manufacturer Web site: *www.safety1st.com*

- Soft Tip Medicine Dispenser by The First Years
  Manufacturer Web site: *www.thefirstyears.com*

I really like medicine droppers because I know I'm giving my child the exact dosage prescribed by my pediatrician.—Sally

○ Tweezers
  Tweezers are needed to remove splinters and ticks. The Clear View Tweezers and Nail Clipper has a magnifier that makes removing splinters and trimming baby's nails easier.
  - Clear View Tweezers and Nail Clipper by Safety 1st
    Manufacturer Web site: *www.safety1st.com*
○ Assortment of Adhesive Bandage Strips
  Have bandages in various sizes and shapes handy for all emergencies. Get the less sticky kind.
  - Children's Adhesive Bandages, Assorted Sizes by Band-Aid, or brand of your choice.
    Vendor Web site: *www.drugstore.com*
○ Gauze Rolls
  To protect open wounds, use gauze rolls ½- to 2-inches wide.
  - Extra Absorbent Rolled Gauze by Johnson & Johnson
    Vendor Web sites: *www.drugstore.com*; *www.walgreens.com*
○ Gauze Pads
  Gauze pads are used for wounds that are too big for Band-Aids.
  - Sterile Gauze Pads, Extra Absorbent 2x2 Inch by Walgreens
  - Sterile Gauze Pads 4x4 Inch by Walgreens
    Vendor Web site: *www.walgreens.com*
○ Adhesive Tape
  Adhesive tape is used to hold gauze pads in place.
  - First-Aid Hurt-Free Tape by Johnson & Johnson
    Vendor Web sites: *www.drugstore.com*; *www.longs.com*
○ Sharp Scissors
  You'll need a pair of sharp scissors for cutting gauze or adhesive tape.
○ Sterile Cotton Balls
  Use sterile cotton balls to clean wounds or apply lotions, creams, or ointments.
  - Cotton Balls by Walgreens
    Vendor Web site: *www.walgreens.com*

- 100% Cotton Balls by Johnson & Johnson
  Vendor Web site: *www.drugstore.com*
○ Cotton Swabs
  Use cotton swabs to apply some medications.
  - Cotton Swabs by Johnson & Johnson
  - Cotton Swabs by Q-Tip
    Vendor Web sites: *www.drugstore.com*; *www.walgreens.com*
○ First-Aid Cold Packs
  Cold packs are used to relieve pain and reduce swelling.
  - Cold Pack Pouch by Sassy
    Manufacturer Web site: *www.sassybaby.com*
  - First-Aid Friends by Munchkin
    Vendor Web sites: *www.babyant.com*; *www.kidsurplus.com*
  - Soft Hug First-Aid Cool Pack by J. L. Childress
    Manufacturer Web site: *www.jlchildress.com*
○ Package of Tongue Depressors
  Keep tongue depressors handy in case you need to make splints for certain injuries. Always consult your doctor before you apply a splint.
○ Small Flashlight and Extra Batteries
  You can use the flashlight to check ears, nose, and throat for redness or inflammation. You can also use it to check pupils for signs of a concussion—or to see in general, when the lights go out.
○ Heating Pad or Hot-Water Bottle
  Some injuries require the use of heat to relieve pain and relax sore muscles. A heating pad or hot-water bottle is great for a colicky tummy. Always consult your pediatrician before you use these items.

I keep a CPR chart on my refrigerator door. Even though you take the class, in an emergency you can forget what to do.—Molly

○ CPR Chart
  Even if you have taken a CPR course, the procedure is easy to forget in an emergency situation. Have the chart handy as a good reminder of the steps to follow in case you need to administer CPR.
○ First-Aid Manual
  The American Red Cross's First-Aid and Safety Handbook gives detailed advice for handling both minor and major emergencies.

Chapter 6

Buying and Packing a Diaper Bag

Choosing the right diaper bag is one of the most important purchasing decisions you'll make. There are several different types of diaper bags on the market. When you are selecting a diaper bag, consider your lifestyle. Do you like to travel lightly or take everything but the kitchen sink? Are you comfortable with a shoulder strap, or would you like a hands-free backpack? Do you plan to carry a separate purse? A smartly designed diaper bag, no matter what style, should keep you well organized and allow you to find what you need in a hurry.

FEATURES TO LOOK FOR

✔ Quality Construction
   Look for sturdy construction, durable fabrics, waterproof linings, and padded shoulder straps/carry handles.

✔ Color
   Consider choosing a bag in a neutral color instead of one of those cute baby prints. Choose one that both parents will be comfortable with. Dad may be taking baby out on his own and may be more comfortable with a stylish, neutral-colored backpack diaper bag.

✔ Multiple Compartments
   A bag with multiple compartments will keep things organized and easy to find.

✔ Two-Way Zippers
   Two-way zippers keep things securely inside and allow for easy access.

✔ Self-Standing Base
   A self-standing base will keep the bag in an upright position no matter where you put it down.

✔ Insulated Side Pockets
These pockets are great for storing bottles and snacks for older babies.

✔ Outside Zippered Pockets
Outside pockets come in handy for keys and other small essentials.

✔ High-Visibility Lining
A light-colored lining on the inside of the bag will make it easier to find what you're looking for.

✔ Snap Hooks
Snap hooks are convenient places to keep baby's pacifier or toys.

✔ Easy-to-Clean Fabric
Fabric should be easy to clean, inside and out, by wiping with a damp cloth.

✔ Classic, Stylish Look
You'll want a bag that can live on after your diaper days are over.

DIAPER BAGS AND BACKPACKS

○ Diaper Bags
  ● Baby Björn Diaper Bag by Baby Björn
    Vendor Web sites: *www.babyage.com*; *www.dreamtimebaby.com*

I love the Baby Björn Diaper Bag! Well worth the price. Lots of room and pockets make it easy to get and stay organized.—Janet

- Do-It-All Diaper Bag by Lands' End
  Manufacturer Web site: *www.landsend.com*
  This diaper bag keeps you organized, with features like a parent pocket to holds sunglasses, cell phone, and other paraphernalia adults require; an adjustable carrying strap makes it easier to tote heavier loads; and the wide-mouth design makes it easy to spot what you need in an instant. The extra-long changing pad cushions baby during changing times.
- Easy Access Overnighter Diaper Bag by One Step Ahead
  Manufacturer Web site: *www.onestepahead.com*
  This diaper bag is roomy enough to handle an overnight trip, yet so well organized you can separate diapers, clothes, and toys. Wide-mouth design gives you easy access to all inside. Big enough for twins.

○ Diaper Backpacks
- Baby Björn Diaper Backpack by Baby Björn
  Vendor Web sites: *www.babybungalow.com*; *www.comfortfirst.com*
- Diaper Backpack by Eddie Bauer
  Manufacturer Web site: *www.eddiebauer.com*
- Backpack Diaper Bag by Lands' End
  Manufacturer Web site: *www.landsend.com*

HOW TO PACK A DIAPER BAG

Packing a diaper bag doesn't take talent; you just have to know what to put in it. Babies need a remarkable amount of stuff to stay comfortable. You should carry certain necessities with you at all times. When you're out with your baby, you want to make sure you have everything with you for any situation that arises. Carrying all the essential items will make life easier and less stressful. Instead of carrying a large purse, put your personal items in a small purse inside the diaper bag. If you have to pass the diaper bag on to Dad, you can easily remove the purse without having to look through the bag to find your things. It's a good idea to keep your diaper bag packed and ready to go. How much you pack of each item will depend on how long you plan to be out. For instance, if you plan to be out for an hour or two, you'll take two to three diapers. If you plan to be out for the whole day, you'll take more. The same rule applies to changes of clothing, food, and drinks. If you go out and use something from the bag, other than food, of course, replace it right away. That way, you'll know the bag's ready to go the next time you leave the house. Use this checklist to make sure your diaper bag is fully stocked for your outings with baby.

NEWBORNS AND INFANTS

○ Diapers
Take more than you think you'll need. Take at least one diaper for every two hours you plan to be out, plus one extra.

❍ Diaper Covers
If you're using cloth diapers, take extra diaper covers.

❍ Diaper Wipes Travel Packs
Small packs of diaper wipes will come in handy for changing dirty diapers and for wiping your own hands. If you don't have a travel-wipes pack, you can put some wipes in a small plastic bag with a zipper seal. The bag will keep them nice and moist until you're ready to use them.
- Natural Care Baby Wipes with Aloe & E, Lightly Scented by Huggies
  Vendor Web site: *www.walgreens.com*
- Quick Wipes by Basic Comfort
  Manufacturer Web site: *www.basiccomfort.com*

❍ Travel Diaper Wipes Warmer
No more cold wipes when traveling about: This portable, fold-and-go pouch keeps wipes warm without batteries, plug-ins, or extension cords. A microwavable insert slips into the pouch and keeps wipes warm for hours. The insert can also be put in the freezer and used as a cold-pack.
- Go Natural Portable Wipes Warmer by Leachco
  Manufacturer Web site: *www.leachco.com*
  Go Natural Portable Wipes Warmer is the safe and convenient way to store all of baby's climate-controlled essentials. A microwavable/freezable insert keeps essentials at the right temperature for hours.
- Travel Wipe Warmer by Dex
  Manufacturer Web site: *www.dexproducts.com*
  The Travel Wipe Warmer's ultraslim design allows you to take it anywhere. Both a home and car adapter are included. Not only great for diaper changes, but also for messy faces and sticky fingers.
- Warm-a-Doodle by Baby Delight
  Manufacturer Web site: *www.babydelight.com*
  This handy diaper tote is designed for carrying the basic essentials for short outings! The reusable gel pack can be heated in seconds to keep wipes warm for hours. The gel pack also doubles as a cool pack, chilling toddlers' favorite snacks and drinks.

❍ Diaper Rash Ointment
You never know when a rash will decide to appear, so you should always have diaper-rash ointment on hand.
- Balmex, Boudreaux's Butt Paste, Desitin, Desitin Creamy
  Vendor Web sites: *www.drugstore.com*; *www.walgreens.com*
- Calendula Cream by California Baby
  Manufacturer Web site: *www.californiababy.com*
- Calendula Baby Cream by Weleda
  Vendor Web site: *www.drugstore.com*

○ Change of Clothes
A change of clothes comes in handy in case baby spits up or the diaper leaks.

- ❏ Onesie
- ❏ Gown, stretch suit, or extra outfit
- ❏ Sweater
- ❏ Hat
- ❏ Booties or socks
- ❏ Receiving blanket
- ❏ Bibs—cloth or disposable
  - Bizzy Bibs by Basic Comfort
    Manufacture Web site: *www.basiccomfort.com*
  - Disposable Bibs by Munchkin
    Manufacturer Web site: *www.munchkininc.com*
  - PeeWee's Disposable Bibs by Continental
    Vendor Web sites: *www.babycatalog.com*; *www.simplybabyandkids.com*
  - Pocket Bibsters Disposable Bibs by Pampers
    Vendor Web sites: *www.longs.com*; *www.walgreens.com*

○ Burp Cloths
Cloth diapers serve nicely as burp cloths. Pack several, especially if you have a baby that spits up frequently.

○ Disposable Dry Washcloths
Use dry washcloths to blot up spills quickly and easily. Each washcloth absorbs up to ten times its weight in water. You can wet these washcloths to wipe little hands, faces, and sensitive bottoms.

- PeeWee's Disposable Dry Washcloths by Continental
  Vendor Web sites: *www.babycatalog.com*; *www.simplybabyandkids.com*

○ Antibacterial Waterless Hand Cleaner
You can use these hand cleaners anywhere, since you don't need water to use them. They come in very handy when you're away from home and you need to clean your hands after changing a dirty diaper or feeding baby.

- Instant Hand Sanitizer with Aloe by Purell
  Vendor Web site: *www.walgreens.com*
- Instant Hand Sanitizer with Moisturizers by Rite Aid
  Vendor Web site: *www.drugstore.com*

○ Plastic Bags
Keep a variety of sizes in your diaper bag for storing dirty diapers, clothes, and shoes. If you prefer, you can buy scented plastic bags for dirty diapers when you are out and about.

Carrying a variety of plastic bags in your diaper bag is a must! By doing so you'll have a place to separate dirty objects from clean ones.—Mary

- Bags on Board Diaper Disposal Bags by Tame Products
  Manufacturer Web site: *www.tameproducts.com*
- Diaper Duck Travel Buddy Dispenser by Munchkin
  Manufacturer Web site: *www.munchkininc.com*
- Diaper Duck Scented Bag Refills by Munchkin
  Manufacturer Web site: *www.munchkininc.com*
- Disposable Diaper Sacks by Sassy
  Manufacturer Web site: *www.sassybaby.com*

○ Disposable Changing Pads

Many diaper bags come with a changing pad, or you can use disposable changing pads. Having a changing pad with you guarantees a clean, sanitary place to lay your baby down, no matter where you are.

- Disposable Changing Pads by Sassy
  Manufacturer Web site: *www.sassybaby.com*
  Multiple-ply Disposable Changing Pads are waterproof, soft, and absorbent. Pads are great for changing, protecting baby from unsanitary conditions and germs, and feeding.
- PeeWee's Disposable Changing Pads by Continental
  Vendor Web site: *www.babycatalog.com*. Search under "Disposable Changing Pads."
  These multiuse pads are great for changing, feeding, or burping your baby.

○ Bottles and Formula

Plan to take enough feedings for the time you're going to be away from home, and one extra in case of delays. If you're using disposable bottles, carry extra disposable bottle bags. There are several ways to carry formula. With the following suggestions, baby will never go hungry when you are away from home.

Bring already-mixed formula and store it in the insulated section of your diaper bag. Or, before you leave the house, fill bottles with the amount of water you'll need, and then add the powdered formula when baby's ready to eat. Carry powdered formula and a scooper from the formula can in a plastic bag with a zipper seal. When baby gets hungry, scoop the right amount of formula into the water and shake. When you are making powdered formula, use one scoop of formula for every 2 ounces of water unless otherwise directed by your pediatrician. If you like, you can buy a formula dispenser that has three sections to store premeasured formula. When you need to mix a bottle, turn the lid to any one of the filled compartments and pour the contents into baby's bottle. Shake the bottle and feed.

- Powder Formula Dispenser & Snack Cup by Avent
  Manufacturer Web site: *www.aventamerica.com*
  The plastic divider keeps the formula separate and ready to mix. The flip-top spout ensures accuracy and prevents messes when pouring. When your baby is ready for solids, use as a handy snack cup by removing the divider.

- Powdered Formula Dispenser by Munchkin
  Manufacturer Web site: *www.munchkininc.com*
  Colorful three-section single-serving containers are ideal for formula or rice cereal. Snap-tight lid and easy-pour spout are great for travel. Removable lid makes cleaning and filling easy.

- Powdered Formula Dispenser by Sassy
  Manufacturer Web site: *www.sassybaby.com*
  The Powdered Formula Dispenser has four single-serving compartments to hold premeasured powdered formula or cereal for meals anytime, anywhere. The snap-on lid keeps powdered formula or cereal fresh and secure during travel.

Some formulas come in premeasured, two-scoop, take-along packs that make 4 ounces of formula. Just add the pack to 4 ounces of water, shake, and feed.

❍ Baby Food and Utensils
  If your baby's on solid foods, be sure to pack a few jars of baby food and a spoon. Planning to be home by baby's mealtime doesn't always work out.

- Safety Spoons by Munchkin
  Manufacturer Web site: *www.munchkininc.com*

- Take & Toss Infant Spoons by The First Years
  Manufacturer Web site: *www.thefirstyears.com*

- Take & Toss Toddler Flatware by The First Years
  Manufacturer Web site: *www.thefirstyears.com*. Search under "Toddler Flatware."

❍ Pacifiers
  Pack several pacifiers in a clean plastic bag. Pacifiers tend to fall on the floor or ground, or get lost between the seats in the car. Having more than one can be a lifesaver.

I keep a pacifier with me at all times. When my baby get fussy it's the only thing that will quiet him down so he can fall asleep.—Jennifer

○ Pacifier Holder

A pacifier holder prevents baby's pacifier from becoming lost. A strap fastener securely holds most pacifiers. A metal clip attaches securely to baby's clothing, car-seat cover, or stroller to hold the pacifier in place—no more fishing around in the car, stroller, or anywhere else for a lost pacifier.

- Clean n' Go by Munchkin
  Manufacturer Web site: *www.munchkininc.com*
- Pacifier & Attacher by The First Years
  Manufacturer Web site: *www.thefirstyears.com*

○ Pacifier Rinser

Dropped pacifiers pick up dirt and germs, so it's important to keep baby's pacifier sparkling clean. Place the dirty pacifier in the spray shield and spritz the dirt away with clean water or antibacterial mouthwash.

- Pacifier Rinser by Prince Lionheart
  Manufacturer Web site: *www.princelionheart.com*

○ Nasal Aspirator

A nasal aspirator is good to have on hand, especially for newborns. If baby spits up through the nose or has a cold, an aspirator will help clear her little nose so she can breathe again.

- Nasal Aspirator by Safety 1st
  Manufacturer Web site: *www.safety1st.com*

○ Medications and Dispenser

Be sure to bring any medications your child may be on, such as Tylenol, antibiotics, Mylicon drops for gas, and so on, as well as a medicine dispenser for administering the medication.

- Medicine Dropper by Safety 1st
  Manufacturer Web site: *www.safety1st.com*

○ Immunization Records

Each time your child is immunized, it will be recorded in your baby's immunization record book. Not only will this booklet keep track of your child's immunizations, but also producing the records will be required when your child starts school.

○ Stain and Odor Removers

Stain and odor removers are great for use when you're away from home. Spots and stains can occur anywhere, and the longer they sit, the harder it is to remove them. Be prepared so you don't have to wait until you get home to treat messes.

- Stain Removing Wipes by Totally Toddler
  Manufacturer Web site: *www.totallytoddler.com*
- Stain and Odor Remover by Mother's Little Miracle
  Vendor Web sites: *www.pottytrainingconcepts.com*; *www.shopplanetkids .com*

○ Snacks and Juice

Have a container of snacks, such as crackers, cereal, or cut-up fruit, handy in case your child gets hungry. Take juice in a bottle, sippy cup, or juice box to wash down the snacks.

○ Disposable Placemats

Disposable placemats instantly create a sanitary, clean, and germ-free eating surface. They're great for restaurants and on tables, counters, and highchairs.

- Table Toppers Placemats by Neat Solutions
  Manufacturer Web site: *www.neatsolutions.com*

○ Tissues

Carry travel-size packages of tissues for runny noses and general cleaning up.

○ Antibiotic Ointments

Once your baby becomes mobile, cuts and scrapes are inevitable. Prevent infection by applying a medicated ointment right away.

- Neosporin First-Aid Antibiotic Ointment
- Polysporin First-Aid Antibiotic Ointment
  Vendor Web sites: *www.drugstore.com; www.longs.com*

○ Band-Aids

Cover wounds to help prevent infection.

- Children's Adhesive Bandages, Assorted Sizes by Band-Aid, or brand of your choice
  Vendor Web site: *www.drugstore.com*

○ Teething Pain Reliever

Pain-relieving gels soothe teething pain. They can be applied every two hours if necessary.

When my baby was teething I brought Baby Fast Teething Pain Relief by Orajel with me wherever I went. It relieves sore gums instantly.—Sandy

- Baby Anbesol by Anbesol
  Manufacturer Web site: *www.anbesol.com*
  Pediatrician-recommended Baby Anbesol works on contact and is alcohol free.
- Baby Orajel Nighttime Formula by Orajel
  Manufacturer Web site: *www.orajel.com*

Baby Orajel Nighttime Formula contains added teething pain reliever for the more intense teething pain that often comes at night; this medicine allows your baby to rest more comfortably.

- Baby Orajel Teething Pain Swabs by Orajel
  Manufacturer Web site: *www.orajel.com*
  Baby Orajel Teething Pain Swabs offer the convenience and portability of the medication and applicator all in one.

- Little Teethers Oral Pain Relief Gel by Little Remedies
  Manufacturer Web site: *www.littleremedies.com*
  Little Teethers Oral Pain Relief Gel is a safe, soothing, easy-to-apply gel that immediately helps to relieve teething pain. Most importantly, this pleasant-tasting topical anesthetic formula is free of alcohol, sugar, saccharin, and artificial dyes.

○ Teething Toys
Chewing on any type of teething toy helps relieve the pain of sore, swollen gums. Cool, water-filled toys are more soothing.

○ Teether Cold Pack
Soothe baby's sore gums when you're on the go. The cooler pocket with reusable ice pack chills the teether and keeps it cold for hours of comfort.

- Teether Cooler by J. L. Childress
  Manufacturer Web site: *www.jlchildress.com*

○ Reusable Cold Packs
If your baby is teething, cold packs are great for keeping water-filled teething toys cold. Store the cold packs in the freezer section of your refrigerator. Just before you leave the house, place the cold packs in one of the insulated sections of your diaper bag, along with the teething toys. Baby will have a nice, cold teether to chew on while you're strolling about. These cold packs are also good for keeping ready-mixed formula cold.

- Reusable Ice Packs by J. L. Childress
  Manufacturer Web site: *www.jlchildress.com*

○ Play Toys
If you're out for any length of time, baby can get bored. Having a few favorite toys with you will help keep baby occupied and entertained.

○ Comfort Object
Bring along a special blanket or toy that baby finds comforting when he gets cranky or tired. It might be just the thing you need to calm him down and send him off to dreamland.

○ Wide-Brimmed Hat
If you are out in the sun, have your baby wear a wide-brimmed hat. Little cheeks and noses get sunburned easily.

○ Sunscreen Lotions
Sunblock protects baby from UVA and UVB rays. Sunscreen lotions should not be used on babies under six months of age.
- Coppertone Water BABIES Spectra3—SPF 50 by Coppertone
  Manufacturer Web site: *www.coppertone.com*
- Everyday/Year-Round Sunscreen Lotion—SPF 30+ by California Baby
  Manufacturer Web site: *www.californiababy.com*

○ Child-Safe Insect Repellent
If you're going to take your baby to the park or any other place where there will be bugs and insects, protect your baby from bites by using a child-safe insect repellent.
- Baby Bug Block by Little Forest
  Vendor Web sites: *www.babyproofingplus.com; www.ourgreenhouse.com*

Baby Bug Block is a wonderful product. When I take my baby outside I don't have to worry about him getting insect or mosquito bites.—Linda

- Citronella Bug Blend SPF 30+ Sunscreen Lotion by California Baby
  Manufacturer Web site: *www.californiababy.com*

THINGS FOR MOM

○ Bottled Water and Snacks
Yes, moms do get hungry and thirsty, too.

○ Nursing Pads, if Breastfeeding
Bring extra nursing pads to prevent leaks and embarrassing stains on your clothes.

○ Extra Shirt
It's nice to have a clean shirt ready in case baby spills or wets.

○ Wallet
Keep some cash in your wallet in case of an emergency.

○ Insurance Card
You may be asked to show your insurance card when you visit the pediatrician, go to a hospital for emergency medical treatment, or when you are buying medication.

○ Cell Phone
Having a cell phone with you allows you to contact someone in case of an emergency or notify your loved ones if you are going to be late.

○ Camera and Film

If you are going someplace special, you will want to catch those precious moments.

○ Index Card

Keep an index card in the diaper bag with your name and phone number on it in case the bag gets lost. If you or the baby get sick or are in an accident, it's a good idea to also have an index card in the bag with the pediatrician's number, your doctor's number, and a number where your spouse, baby's grandparents, or a neighbor can be reached.

I know this sounds like a lot of stuff to carry around with you, but it's better to be prepared. You're probably wondering how everything is going to fit into one diaper bag, but—it does!

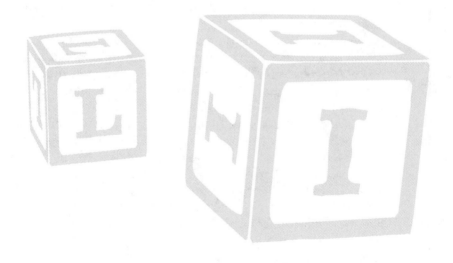

Chapter 7

How to Find and Interview a Nanny

We all want responsible, dependable professionals to care for our children, but finding a good nanny is not always an easy task. The process takes patience and a lot of research to find just the right person. You want to hire someone who truly enjoys taking care of children and is in the field for all the right reasons. In this chapter, you'll find the important guidelines you need for keeping your children safe and happy with a nanny.

FINDING A NANNY

The first step in the process of finding a nanny is to ask yourself a few key questions:

What would my ideal nanny be like? The type of nanny you hire will depend on your own situation. Do you work in or out of the house? Are you a stay-at-home mom? Do you need a full-time nanny, someone that comes part-time every day, or someone that comes in a few times a week? Do you want an older, mature person with a lot of experience, or would you prefer a younger, more energetic person? Make a list of traits and qualities to refer to when you start interviewing applicants or talking to nanny agencies.

When should I start looking for a nanny? If you plan to take some time off from work after the baby is born, you don't have to start looking for a nanny until after the baby arrives. If you try to hire the nanny too far in advance, she may not hold the time slot open for you. If you plan to go back to work right away, start looking around your seventh month so you'll have a nanny lined up before the baby is born. In either case, be sure to leave yourself a time cushion because finding the perfect person for your family might take a while.

Before hiring a nanny, I sat down and made a list of questions to ask each candidate during the interview.—Melanie

There are a number of great ways to find a nanny:

1. *Use word of mouth*: Have friends and family ask around about nannies who might be available. Sometimes a friend has a nanny whom she or he is ready to let go of because the children are older and will be in school most of the time. Sometimes a mother or father decides not to work anymore, to stay home and take care of the kids. This is the ideal way to find a nanny because you're familiar with the family she's worked for and you know her references will be reliable.

2. *Advertise in mothers' and twins' club newsletters*: Placing an ad in a local newsletter will help you find someone qualified. And nannies looking for work by advertising in these newsletters will most likely have references from various members in the club.

3. *Go to online Web sites* such as *www.4nannies.com* and *www.nanny network.com*. They offer some of the same services as nanny-placement agencies, and at a much lower cost.

4. *Post an ad at a local college*: Many students are looking for nanny positions to help pay their way through school.

5. *Post an ad at local churches or synagogues*: This is a good route if you're looking for someone part time and inexpensive. You may

find a grandma-type who would love to spend time with your children while making a little extra money.

6. *Call a local job-resource center*: They may have a list of people seeking nanny positions, or be able to refer you to another agency.

7. *Call the local nanny-placement agencies in your area*: The agencies will do the searching and some of the screening for you. They will do their best to find candidates that meet your needs. Most agencies also verify a nanny's work experience, do a background check to see whether she has a criminal record, and check her driving record. The agency may also require blood and tuberculosis tests and proof of a recent physical checkup from job candidates to make sure that the nanny is in good health. The one drawback about finding a nanny through an agency is that you have to pay a hefty fee. However, if that's the only way you can find a person you trust with your children, it may be well worth the cost.

8. *Place an ad in the newspaper*: Consider this a last resort, as you'll probably get lots of calls, and screening will be difficult. Instead of answering the phone each time it rings, put an outgoing message on your answering machine asking potential candidates to leave their name, phone number, and the names and phone numbers of their references. That way, you can check references before deciding whom you want to interview.

INTERVIEWING A NANNY

The prospect of inviting a stranger into your home to care for your child, your most precious gift, can be overwhelming. There are many questions you need to ask to find safe, quality care for your child. It makes sense to find out as much as possible about a prospective nanny well before the first day of employment.

First, check references. Ask each nanny you're considering for a list of past and present references. Be sure to call and talk to each person on the list. Ask former employers specific questions. Don't ask vague questions like whether or not they liked the nanny. Instead, ask for details such as what exactly they liked about her, and what they disliked. Also ask them to describe her strengths and weaknesses.

While you're interviewing the nanny, communicate your needs and expectations. You'll want her beliefs about child rearing to align with yours so your children won't be confused by different rules and routines. Offer her scenarios and see how she responds. For instance, ask her, "What would you do if the baby wouldn't stop crying or wouldn't go to sleep?" "How would you handle a dispute between two siblings?" "What form of discipline do you believe in?" Listen carefully to her answers, both what she says and what she implies. Above all, look for common sense; you want someone who can think quickly, clearly, and rationally when handling any situation that arises.

Talk about salary and benefits, map out an accurate work schedule, and work on establishing household rules and boundaries everyone can respect. Make it clear that any ill feelings or disputes on either side should be brought out in the open and discussed before problems get out of hand and things become uncomfortable for both parties. If she will be driving your child, ask for a copy of her driving record.

Hire a person who has experience taking care of children the same age as yours. If you have a newborn and she has only taken care of toddlers, you may want to consider someone else. Let the prospective nanny spend some time with your children while she's in your home interviewing. Observe how she interacts with your children and how your children respond to her.

After you have hired the perfect nanny, have her start working well in advance of when you go back to work. Ease her in slowly. Teach her the routine you want her to follow. After a few days, let her take over as if you weren't there. Observe how she handles herself and the children throughout the day. If everything goes well and you are satisfied with your choice, you can go back to work feeling that your children are in good hands. If for some reason you're not happy with the nanny, don't hesitate to let her go and find another. Your children's welfare is the most important thing.

Your children are your most precious possessions. Make sure you check each candidate's references thoroughly.—Jackie

Name _____

_____

Address _____

_____

Phone Number _____

_____

Experience

1. Why did you become a nanny?

_____

_____

2. How long have you been a nanny?

_____

_____

3. What do you like about being a nanny?

_____

_____

4. Where have you worked before?

_____

_____

5. What is the age range of the children you have cared for?

_____

_____

6. Why did you leave your last position?

_____

_____

7. What are some of the rules you've followed in other households that you think work well?

_____

_____

8. What sorts of rules don't work for you?

_____

_____

9. Is there anything in particular that makes it difficult for you to work with certain parents or children?

_____

_____

Education

1. Do you have any formal early childhood development education or childcare training?

_____

_____

2. Do you have CPR and children's first-aid training? May I see your certification card? (If it isn't current, ask her to get recertified. If she can't take the class on her own, you may offer to send her and pick up the expense.)

_____

_____

Logistics

1. Are you looking for a live-in or live-out position?

_____

_____

2. Do you have any health problems that might interfere with your job?

_____

_____

3. What hours are you looking for?

_____

_____

4. When can you start working?

_____

_____

5. Do you drive? Do you have a current driver's license?

_____

_____

6. How will you get to work? Do you have your own car, or will you be taking public transportation?

_____

_____

7. Are you willing to do any light housework such as laundry, dishes, or straightening up while the baby is sleeping?

_____

_____

8. Can you work evenings or weekends?

_____

_____

9. Will you be available to travel with our family for weekends/vacations?

_____

_____

10. What is your salary range, and when and how do you like to be paid?

_____

_____

Rules and Beliefs
Please specify your feelings about:
1. Smoking

_____

_____

2. Drinking

_____

_____

3. Use of telephone

_____

_____

4. Food (What would you like us to have for you to eat and drink?)

_____

_____

5. Television

_____

_____

Approach to Child Rearing
Newborns and Infants
1. How would you pacify a baby if she woke up before it was time to eat?

_____

_____

2. Do you believe in picking a baby up every time he cries, or do you let him cry it out?

_____

_____

3. What method do you use to get a baby to sleep?

_____

_____

4. How would you console a crying baby?

_____

_____

Toddlers and Older Children

1. In your opinion, what is the most important thing to be aware of while taking care of my children? (The safety of the children should be included in her answer. This issue applies to children of all ages.)

_____

_____

2. How would you keep my child entertained throughout the day?

_____

_____

3. What would you do if my child threw a tantrum?

_____

_____

4. (If you have more than one child) How would you handle a disagreement between two of my children?

_____

_____

5. If my child needed to be disciplined, what method would you use? (If she states any form of discipline that doesn't fit in with your beliefs, she's out of there.)

_____

_____

6. What might a typical day with my child be like?

_____

_____

How Would You Handle These Emergency Situations?

1. What would you do if my child became sick or got hurt?

2. If a baby in your care spit up and started choking, what would you do?

3. When and how do you use a bulb syringe?

Your Opinion of the Candidate

1. Was she pleasant?

2. Did she answer all your questions to your satisfaction?

3. Did she seem comfortable with the children?

4. Did the children seem to like her?

5. While you are away from the house, will you feel comfortable knowing your children are at home with her?

CANDIDATE'S LIST OF REFERENCES

Name ——————————— Phone Number ———————

Start Date ——————————— Why You Left Position ————

Ages of Children ——————————————————————

Comments ———————————————————————————

——————————————————————————————————

——————————————————————————————————

Name ——————————— Phone Number ———————

Start Date ——————————— Why You Left Position ————

Ages of Children ——————————————————————

Comments ———————————————————————————

——————————————————————————————————

——————————————————————————————————

Name ——————————— Phone Number ———————

Start Date ——————————— Why You Left Position ————

Ages of Children ——————————————————————

Comments ———————————————————————————

——————————————————————————————————

——————————————————————————————————

Name ——————————— Phone Number ———————

Start Date ——————————— Why You Left Position ————

Ages of Children ——————————————————————

Comments ———————————————————————————

——————————————————————————————————

——————————————————————————————————

Name ——————————— Phone Number ———————

Start Date ——————————— Why You Left Position ————

Ages of Children ——————————————————————

Comments ———————————————————————————

——————————————————————————————————

——————————————————————————————————

Chapter 8
Childproofing Your Home

It's never too early to childproof your home. Little babies grow quickly. Before you know it, they'll be crawling all over the house and getting into everything. Inspect every room in your house for possible hazards. To get a child's-eye view of each room, crouch down on your hands and knees, and also roll onto your back. Check out everything that would be within your child's reach when he's crawling and begins to stand up and walk. It is best to do all your childproofing in one fell swoop. Doing this will ensure that, as your child grows, he won't encounter a hazard that's been left exposed.

There are many childproofing products on the market that will help make your home a safe environment for your baby. Installing these products will give you peace of mind knowing you've done your best to protect your little one from dangers both obvious and hidden.

CRIB SAFETY TIPS

Babies spend a lot of time in bed. Your child's crib should be as safe as possible, especially if she's at an age to be left alone to nap or sleep.

✔ Use tightly fitting crib sheets. Baby can become entangled in loose crib sheets that pull away from the mattress.

✔ Keep the mattress at the proper level according to your baby's age and capabilities. A crib mattress for a newborn can be placed at the highest level. When your child can sit up or pull up to a standing position, the mattress should be placed at the lowest level in the crib.

✔ Keep side rails up at all times for newborns and babies.

✔ Remove crib bumpers if baby crawls under them or tries to stand on them.

✔ If you have a toddler who's ready to climb out of the crib, lower the side rail. If he does try to climb out and falls in the process, he will be closer to the floor.

✔ Never put a pillow or stuffed animals in the crib.

CRIB SAFETY PRODUCTS

○ Crib Teething Rails
Teething babies often chew on their crib's railing. Teething rails keep baby's teeth safe and soothe tender gums. And they keep the crib looking nice!

- Crib Rail Teether by Prince Lionheart
Vendor Web site: *www.safeandsecurebaby.com*

- Easy Teether Crib Rail Cover by Leachco
Manufacturer Web site: *www.leachco.com*

○ Crib Tent
A crib tent keeps baby from falling or climbing out of bed, keeps pets out of baby's bed, and keeps toys and bottles in.

- Cozy Crib Tent by Tots in Mind
Manufacturer Web site: *www.totsinmind.com*

GENERAL FURNITURE SAFETY TIPS

As soon as your baby learns to pull himself up and climb, furniture is the biggest hazard. To prevent serious injury to your child, you will want to take the necessary precautions.

✔ Using furniture straps or bolts, anchor bookshelves, dressers, tables, TV sets, and anything else a child might pull on top of himself.

✔ Test furniture by putting your weight on lower shelves or pulling out the top drawers and leaning on them. If there's any hint that they'll tip forward, anchor them to a wall or keep the room off-limits with a safety gate.

✔ Cover sharp-edged furniture with corner guards to prevent serious injury.

GENERAL FURNITURE SAFETY PRODUCTS

○ Corner Guards, Standard Size
Learning to stand up and walk means baby will be taking lots of falls. Covering sharp furniture corners with padded guards can mean the difference between a mild "ouchie" and a major injury.

- Cushiony Corner Guards by Prince Lionheart
  Manufacturer Web site: *www.princelionheart.com*
  Four Cushiony Corner Guards easily adhere to sharp corners. Full-length double-stick tape keeps corner guards securely fastened and removes quickly and easily when no longer needed.

- Furniture Corner Cushions by Safety 1st
  Manufacturer Web site: *www.safety1st.com*
  Furniture Corner Cushions are soft and rounded to help protect children from sharp corners. Clear design blends in with furniture.

- Soft Corner Protector by Kidco
  Manufacturer Web site: *www.kidco.com*
  The super soft, gel-like corner helps protect your child from sharp edges, and the ribbed design provides more flexibility. Adhesive mount leaves no marks upon removal.

○ Corner Guards, Jumbo Size
Jumbo corner guards provide extra cushioning for maximum coverage.

- Jumbo Corner Guard by Prince Lionheart
  Manufacturer Web site: *www.princelionheart.com*

○ Table Edge Guards
Protect both round and square tables that have sharp, hard edges. To determine the appropriate size guard for your table, add the total length of all sides in inches or centimeters.

- Expandable Table Edge Bumper by Safety 1st
  Manufacturer Web site: *www.safety1st.com*

- Jumbo Edge Guard by Prince Lionheart
  Manufacturer Web site: *www.princelionheart.com*

- Table Edge Guard by Prince Lionheart
  Manufacturer Web site: *www.princelionheart.com*

○ Furniture Anchors
Secure furniture to the wall to help prevent tipping.

- Anti-Tip Furniture Strap by Kidco
  Manufacturer Web site: *www.kidco.com*
- Furniture Brackets by Mommy's Helper
  Vendor Web sites: *www.babybungalow.com*; *www.babyuniverse.com*

Mommy's Helper brackets are easy to install and keep furniture in place. I don't have to worry about anything tipping over on my child.—Alice

- Furniture Wall Straps by Safety 1st
  Manufacturer Web site: *www.safety1st.com*

○ TV Guard
  A TV Guard keeps curious little fingers away from television controls, yet it's transparent, so remote controls remain operable for parents.
  - TV Guard by Parent Units
    Manufacturer Web site: *www.parentunits.com*
  - TV Guard for Large Televisions by Parent Units
    Manufacturer Web site: *www.parentunits.com*
  - TV Guard for Flat Screen by Parent Units
    Manufacturer Web site: *www.parentunits.com*

○ VCR Locks
  Use VCR locks to prevent children from inserting objects into the cassette opening of your VCR.
  - VCR Guard by Parent Unit
    Manufacturer Web site: *www.parentunits.com*
  - Child Safe VCR Lock by Safety 1st
    Vendor Web site: *www.safetycentral.com*

○ DVD Guard
  A DVD guard is a clear plastic shield that stops babies from pushing buttons; it can help prevent damage to your valuable equipment.
  - DVD Guard by Parent Units
    Manufacturer Web site: *www.parentunits.com*

BATHROOM SAFETY TIPS

The bathroom can be a hazardous place for your child. Here are some simple childproofing tips:

✔ Install locks on all toilets to prevent children from drowning accidentally, and to keep them from dropping objects into the water.

✔ Place a hook-and-eye lock or a sliding lock beyond a child's reach on the bathroom door, and keep it secured when you're not using the bathroom.

✔ Remove sharp objects and appliances such as hair dryers and curling irons from counters to protect children from injury and electrical shock.

✔ Cover all electrical plugs, whether used or unused.

✔ Keep all medications, toiletries, and cleaning products in original containers and in a locked closet, cabinet, or drawer.

✔ Install safety latches on all cabinets and drawers.

✔ Set hot-water heaters no higher than 120 degrees to prevent accidental scalding. Always check the water temperature with a thermometer to make sure it's not too hot for your children.

✔ Place a nonslip mat in the bathtub to prevent falls.

✔ Put a faucet cover over the bathtub spout to protect your child's head.

✔ Make sure you can open the bathroom door from either side in case it becomes locked accidentally.

✔ Never leave your child unattended while in the bathtub—not even for a minute.

✔ Teach your child to stay seated in the bathtub at all times.

✔ Install a night light in the bathroom.

BATHROOM SAFETY PRODUCTS

○ Toilet Lid Locks
Keep curious little ones out of the toilet bowl by locking the lid. Babies love water, and splashing in the toilet can be lots of fun. It's also very dangerous. When babies lean into a toilet bowl, they may lose their balance, fall forward, and drown in as little as one inch of water.

- Cover Clamp Toilet Lock by Safety 1st
  Manufacturer Web site: *www.safety1st.com*
  This lock helps keep toilet cover closed to curious children, but it unlocks easily for adults. It's easy to install, with no tools required.

- Lid Lock by Mommy's Helper
  Vendor Web site: *www.babycenter.com*
  Quick and easy to open. The one-hand release operation is easy for an adult hand, but difficult for a child. It easily attaches to all types of bowls and lids, and it's simple to remove when not needed. No adhesive is required, and you don't have to unbolt the seat to install.

- Toilet Lock by Kidco
  Manufacturer Web site: *www.kidco.com*
  The Toilet Lock can be used on thick, padded, or fabric-covered toilet seats. The arm is height adjustable to accommodate thicker toilet seat

covers. It automatically resets when the lid is lowered. Out-of-the-way placement means it is easy to clean.

The Toilet Lock by Kidco costs more than others but it's so worth it. It's easy to use and closes by itself when you lower the lid. —Cynthia

○ Bath Thermometers
Prevent accidental scalding by using a bath thermometer that measures the actual temperature of the water and indicates the ideal range for your baby's bath.
  - Bath Pal Thermometer by Safety 1st
    Manufacturer Web site: *www.safety1st.com*
  - Safety Bath Ducky by Munchkin
    Manufacturer Web site: *www.munchkininc.com*

○ Heat-Warning Bath Cradles
Heat-warning bath inserts create a warm, comfortable, and secure bathing environment. A safety disc turns white when water is too hot for baby. These inserts are ideal for bathing infants in sinks, baby baths, and on the counter.
  - Safety Baby Bath Cradle by Munchkin
    Manufacturer Web site: *www.munchkininc.com*

○ Heat Warning Bath Mat
Appliqués and bath mats will warn you when the water is too hot for your baby.
  - Tub-Rug Jr. by Kel-Gar
    Manufacturer Web site: *www.kelgar.com*

○ Slip-Resistant Bathmats
Nonskid, textured bathmats prevent slipping and falling in the bathtub. They adhere securely to the tub floor and ensure that children always feel stable in the bath.
  - Surf Friends Bathtub Mat by Munchkin
    Manufacturer Web site: *www.munchkininc.com*

○ Spout Covers
Making bath time safer, soft spout covers guard the entire faucet to protect children from accidental bumps and burns.
  - Faucet Friends by Kel-Gar
    Manufacturer Web site: *www.kelgar.com*
  - Soft Spout Cover by Safety 1st
    Manufacturer Web site: *www.safety1st.com*

- Super Soft Spout Guard by Sassy
  Manufacturer Web site: *www.sassybaby.com*
○ Transitional Bathtubs
  Place a transitional bathtub inside an adult-sized bathtub, and baby will feel more comfortable and secure. Transitional tubs make bath time easier whether you are at home or traveling.
  - Bath 'N Bumper by Leachco
    Manufacturer Web site: *www.leachco.com*
  - Snug-Tub by Kel-Gar (also comes in Deluxe and Jr.)
    Manufacturer Web site: *www.kelgar.com*

I love the Snug Tub! It makes the big bathtub a much softer area for my daughter to sit in.—Monica

○ Transitional Bathtub with White Hot Safety Disc
  The Inflatable Safety Duck Tub is an inflatable, padded tub with a White Hot safety disc that reveals the word "hot" when the water is too hot for baby.
  - Inflatable Safety Duck Tub by Munchkin
    Manufacturer Web site: *www.munchkininc.com*
○ Tub Side Knee and Elbow Savers for Parents
  These protectors let you enjoy greater comfort while you are bathing your baby. They protect your knees and elbows while you lean over the tub.
  - Sit & Store Tub Side Seat by The First Years
    Vendor Web sites: *www.babiesrus.com*; *www.onestepahead.com*
  - Tubside Kneeler & Step Stool by Safety 1st
    Manufacturer Web site: *www.safety1st.com*

The Tubside Kneeler & Step Stool provides cushioning for your elbows and knees and lessens the strain on your back while bathing your baby.—Janet

○ Splash Guard
  Children can become rambunctious during bath time. Keep water in the tub, not on the floor, to prevent slipping and water damage.
  - Splash Guard by Basic Comfort
    Manufacturer Web site: *www.basiccomfort.com*

○ Spray Attachment for Bath or Sink
A spray attachment makes it easier to shampoo and rinse baby's hair without getting water in his face. The sprayer attaches easily to bath or sink faucets.
  • Bath Shower Spray by Sassy
    Manufacturer Web site: *www.sassybaby.com*
○ Bath Visors
During bath time, visors help keep shampoo away from baby's face.
  • Bath and Sun Visors by Sassy
    Manufacturer Web site: *www.sassybaby.com*
  • Sudsy Sun Shield Shampoo and Sun Visor by Kel-Gar
    Manufacturer Web site: *www.kelgar.com*
○ Toy Bags
Keep your bathroom tidy by storing bath toys in a bag. Toy bags mount securely, with suction cups that are easy to install and quick to remove, to any smooth surface.
  • Bath Toy Bag by Safety 1st
    Manufacturer Web site: *www.safety1st.com*
  • Large Tub Toy Organizer by Sassy
    Manufacturer Web site: *www.sassybaby.com*
  • Tub Toy Organizer by Sassy
    Manufacturer Web site: *www.sassybaby.com*
  • Sudsy Storage Tub Toy Holder/Organizer by Kel-Gar
    Manufacturer Web site: *www.kelgar.com*
○ Night Lights
If you have to make a trip to the bathroom during the night, these lights will show you the way. The Auto-Sensor Night Light automatically turns on in the dark.
  • Auto-Sensor Night Light by Safety 1st
    Manufacturer Web site: *www.safety1st.com*
  • Dim 'n Bright Auto Sensor Night Light by Safety 1st
    Manufacturer Web site: *www.safety1st.com*

KITCHEN SAFETY TIPS

Many dangers lurk in the average kitchen. Because you probably spend a lot of time in the kitchen, you'll want to make it as safe as possible. Here's how:

✔ Keep children away from the stovetop at all times.

✔ Keep children away from stove knobs at all times.

✔ Never cook while children are playing near the stove, and never leave hot pots and pans unattended.

✔ Always keep handles of pots and pans turned toward the back of the stove. Whenever possible, use the back burners for cooking.

✔ Keep ovens and microwave doors locked if possible.

✔ Store glasses and precious china in a locked cabinet or on a high shelf, out of reach.

✔ Keep knives and other sharp tools, such as electric mixer blades, in latched drawers.

✔ Keep all cleaning products and medicines in original containers (so that there's no mistaking what they are), and store them in a locked closet, cabinet, or drawer.

✔ Store trash in a locked cabinet or closet.

✔ Place all plug-in appliances away from children's reach, and cover electrical plugs not in use.

KITCHEN SAFETY PRODUCTS

○ Appliance Locks
Keep your child from opening the oven and other kitchen appliances with these easy-to-use appliance locks.

● Fridge Guard by Parent Units
Manufacturer Web site: *www.parentunits.com*
Children love to open and close refrigerator doors. The Fridge Guard appliance safety latch keeps them safe and shut.

● Multi-Purpose Appliance Latch by Safety 1st
Manufacturer Web site: *www.safety1st.com*
Ideal for the freezer, refrigerator, microwave, and dishwasher! The secure press-and-pull lock helps keep appliances closed.

● On-Off Appliance Lock by Kidco
Manufacturer Web site: *www.kidco.com*
The On-Off Appliance Lock can be used on refrigerators, freezers, and ovens. The on-off feature is exclusively adult controlled. This tool automatically locks when in the "on" position.

● Oven Lock by Safety 1st
Manufacturer Web site: *www.safety1st.com*
This secure lock helps keep the oven door closed to children. This heat-resistant lock is easy for adults to use and install.

○ Stove Knob Covers
To prevent burns and dangerous gas leaks, keep busy little hands from turning the knobs on your stove.

● Stove Knob Covers by Safety 1st
Manufacturer Web site: *www.safety1st.com*

○ Stove Guards
Protect your child from hot burners and pans with stove guards. They ensure that only an adult can access the stove.

- Stove Guard by Prince Lionheart
  Manufacturer Web site: *www.princelionheart.com*
- Stove Top Shield by Safety 1st
  Vendor Web site: *www.safeandsecurebaby.com*

CABINET AND DRAWER SAFETY TIPS

Children love playing in cabinets and drawers. Don't underestimate your child's curiosity—even cabinets that you think are out of reach can be hazardous. Follow these tips:

✔ Lock all cabinets and drawers that contain medications, poisons, sharp objects, and other dangerous items.

✔ Don't forget to lock cabinets that are above countertops.

✔ Use cabinet and drawer locks in every room in the house.

CABINET AND DRAWER SAFETY PRODUCTS

○ Cabinet and Drawer Latches and Locks
- Adhesive Mount Drawer & Cabinet Lock by Kidco
  Manufacturer Web site: *www.kidco.com*
  This is the only lock that mounts without tools, holes, or screws. It's perfect for use on stereo equipment, glass, metal, and mirrored surfaces.
- Cabinet & Drawer Spring Latches by Safety 1st
  Manufacturer Web site: *www.safety1st.com*
  The "spring-loaded" feature makes these locks longer lasting and more durable.
- Cabinet Slide Lock by Safety 1st
  Manufacturer Web site: *www.safety1st.com*
  These child-resistant locks work on cabinets with handles or knobs.
- Double Locks by Safety 1st
  Manufacturer Web site: *www.safety1st.com*
  This double lock allows a cabinet or drawer to open only 1½ inches.
- Lazy Susan Cabinet Lock by Safety 1st
  Manufacturer Web site: *www.safety1st.com*
  These Lazy Susan Cabinet Locks help keep children out of revolving corner cabinets that don't have handles.
- Secure Slide Cabinet Lock by Safety 1st
  Manufacturer Web site: *www.safety1st.com*
  This lock helps keep children out of cabinets and has a one-handed slide release for parents.

- Tot Lok Deluxe Starter Set by Safety 1st
  Manufacturer Web site: *www.safety1st.com*. Search under "Tot Lok."
  This is a patented magnetic locking system for cabinet drawers and
  doors; it works with the Tot Lok Magnetic Key.

The Tot Lok is the best product I have found to keep my children out of my cabinets. Kids can't open cabinets even a crack without the key.—Mary

- Ultra Secure Cabinet & Drawer Latches by Safety 1st
  Manufacturer Web site: *www.safety1st.com*
  These latches are spring loaded for extra durability; they conveniently
  fold down for periods of nonuse.

ELECTRICAL SAFETY TIPS

Small children are tempted to play with anything within their reach. Electrical
outlets in most homes are at just the right height to attract crawling babies
and toddlers. Here are some electrical safety tips:

✔ To protect your child from electrocution or shock, all electrical outlets
  that are not in use should be covered using outlet plugs.

✔ Cover all electrical outlets and power strips that are in use. The products
  listed below correspond to each type of electrical outlet.

✔ All electrical cords should be shortened so that children cannot get tangled or shocked, and cannot pull appliances down on top of themselves.

✔ Move all fans out of the reach of children.

ELECTRICAL SAFETY PRODUCTS

○ Outlet Plugs and Caps
  *Keep children from putting fingers or small objects into the sockets using
  outlet plugs and caps.*

  - Deluxe Press-Fit Outlet Plugs by Safety 1st
    Manufacturer Web site: *www.safety1st.com*

  - Electrical Outlet Caps by Kidco
    Manufacturer Web site: *www.kidco.com*

  - Outlet Plugs by Safety 1st
    Manufacturer Web site: *www.safety1st.com*

  - Ultra Clear Outlet Plugs by Safety 1st
    Manufacturer Web site: *www.safety1st.com*

- Outlet Covers
  These items automatically cover the outlet when the plug is removed, and you don't have to pry a cap off when you want to use the outlet.
  - Double-Touch Plug 'N Outlet Covers by Safety 1st
    Manufacturer Web site: *www.safety1st.com*
  - Standard Outlet Cover by Kidco
    Manufacturer Web site: *www.kidco.com*

These Kidco Outlet Covers are the absolute best! They are functional past toddlerhood.—Sandy

  - Swivel Outlet Cover by Safety 1st
    Manufacturer Web site: *www.safety1st.com*
  - Two-Touch Outlet Covers by Safety 1st
    Manufacturer Web site: *www.safety1st.com*
- Power Strip Covers
  These items cover the entire power strip, including the on/off switch.
  - Power Strip Cover by Safety 1st
    Manufacturer Web site: *www.safety1st.com*
  - Power Strip Safety Cover by Mommy's Helper
    Vendor Web sites: *www.babycatalog.com*; *www.safeandsecurebaby.com*
- Cord Shortener
  Cord shorteners keep dangling power cords safely out of a child's reach. They neatly wind up any loose cord to prevent a tripping accident and to keep children from pulling lamps and appliances off tables and counters.
  - Cord Shortener by Safety 1st
    Manufacturer Web site: *www.safety1st.com*
  - Outlet Cover with Cord Shortener by Safety 1st
    Manufacturer Web site: *www.safety1st.com*

DOOR SAFETY TIPS

Be sure to prevent your child from getting into off-limits rooms and closets. Follow these tips:

✔ Install doorknob covers on doors that you don't want children to open.

✔ While you're closing doors, watch for little fingers. Use finger guards to prevent your child's fingers from getting crushed.

✔ Your child can be hurt if she mistakes a sliding glass door for an open doorway. Prevent accidents with decals placed at your child's eye level.

○ Doorknob Covers
Slip doorknob covers over household doorknobs to protect children from leaving the house or going into rooms that are off-limits.

- Door Knob Covers by Mommy's Helper
  Vendor Web sites: *www.babybungalow.com*; *www.netkidswear.com*
- Door Knob Lock by Kidco
  Manufacturer Web site: *www.kidco.com*

○ Door Stops and Positioners
Use door stops and positioners to prevent doors from slamming shut. Slide the door positioner under the door, which will then stay put.

- Door Positioner by Kidco
  Manufacturer Web site: *www.kidco.com*
- Soft Jamb Door Stop by Kidco
  Manufacturer Web site: *www.kidco.com*

○ Finger Guards
Finger guards keep doors from closing completely, helping prevent painful and serious finger injuries.

- Finger Guard by Kidco
  Manufacturer Web site: *www.kidco.com*
  The Finger Guard fits most interior and exterior doors. It keeps doors from slamming on little fingers, and helps prevent painful and serious finger injuries.
- Finger Pinch Guard by Safety 1st
  Manufacturer Web site: *www.safety1st.com*
  This safety aid can prevent children from pinching their fingers in doors. The soft, flexible material prevents doors from closing all the way.
- On/Off Door Finger Protector by Kid
  Vendor Web sites: *www.babyant.com*; *www.childsafetystore.com*
  This product automatically engages when in the active position, and cannot accidentally lock when the door is closed. The Finger Protector's soft, flexible material is harmless to doors and woodwork. There is an adult-controlled on/off feature.

○ Folding Door Locks
These locks keep children from opening folding doors. They are used most often for laundry rooms, closets, and garbage areas.

- Bi-Fold Door Lock by Safety 1st
  Manufacturer Web site: *www.safety1st.com*
- Slid-Lok by Mommy's Helper
  Vendor Web site: *www.babyuniverse.com*

○ French Door Locks
These special locks lock one side of a door, allowing access from the other side. They automatically reset after use.

- Door Lever Lock by Kidco
  Manufacturer Web site: *www.kidco.com*
- Lever Handle Lock by Safety 1st
  Manufacturer Web site: *www.safety1st.com*

○ Sliding Door Locks
Use sliding door locks to lock all doors that lead outside, especially if you have a swimming pool. Use locks on glass, mirrors, wood, and other surfaces where drilling is impractical.

- Sliding Door Lock by Kidco
  Manufacturer Web site: *www.kidco.com*

SAFETY GATES

Once your child is mobile, she is ready for action. This is the time to put up safety gates. Safety gates are an invaluable aid in childproofing your home. No matter which area you want off-limits to your child, there's a gate that will help you. From hallway gates to gates that fit at the top and bottom of a stairway, these items give you control over which rooms your child can visit.

Buy gates before your child is six months old to guarantee that you will have them in place before he starts crawling. If you have a multilevel house, remember that babies can pull themselves up stairs before they start walking. There are three basic safety-gate designs: pressure-mounted gates, hardware-mounted gates, and customizable gates.

○ Pressure-Mounted Gates
These gates require no hardware, relying on pressure to stay in place. They're the easiest, least expensive choice, although they are not as secure as hardware-mounted gates.

- Center Gateway Model G15 by Kidco
  Manufacturer Web site: *www.kidco.com*
  The U-shaped frame of this gate remains firmly installed while the center walk-through door can open easily in either direction. The gate expands from 29¼ inches to 37½ inches wide and stands 29½ inches tall.
- Easy-Fit Security Gate by Safety 1st
  Manufacturer Web site: *www.safety1st.com*
  The Easy-Fit Security Gate comes equipped with a memory feature to make reinstallation fast and simple. The gate expands from 28 inches to 42 inches, and stands 27 inches tall.

- Lift and Lock Security Gate by Safety 1st
  Manufacturer Web site: *www.safety1st.com*
  The Lift and Lock Security Gate is easy to operate because all the controls are located in the handle. Simply raise the complete-control top handle and switch between adjust, lock, and release modes as needed. This gate can be pressure mounted in standard entryways, or mounted with hardware in entryways or at the top of the stairs.
- SimpleEffort Gate by Evenflo
  Manufacturer Web site: *www.evenflo.com*
  This electronic gate is easy to open with the touch of a button and then a slight push on the gate. The red/green indicator shows whether the gate is properly locked. The door swings open for easy walk-through. This gate is designed for use at bottom of stairs and doorways.

○ Hardware-Mounted Gates
  These gates mount to the surrounding walls or furniture with hardware. Although they are more expensive and harder to install, hardware-mounted gates are much sturdier than models that rely on pressure.

- All Clear Swing Gate by The First Years
  Manufacturer Web sites: *www.babyuniverse.com*; *www.walmart.com*
  Because toddlers often try to climb up and over standard gates, this gate is designed with kid-tough clear panels that are free of footholds. The gate can be hardware- or pressure-mounted. The gate expands from 27½ inches to 42½ inches wide and is 30 inches tall.
- Angle-Mount Wood Safeway Model G32 by Kidco
  Manufacturer Web site: *www.kidco.com*
  The Wood Safeway gate has hardware that lets you install the gate in any position, including at angled banisters and walls. The gate stands 31 inches high, which makes a great barrier for both children and pets.
- Safeway Model G20 by Kidco
  Manufacturer Web site: *www.kidco.com*
  This is the top-rated wall-mount, swinging gate. It is the only expandable, plastic-coated, steel gate available that is 30½ inches high. This gate is recommended for use at the top of stairs and as a window barrier. It expands from openings 24¾ inches wide to 43½ inches wide.
- SimpleEffort Plus Gate by Evenflo
  Manufacturer Web site: *www.evenflo.com*
  This electronic gate is similar to the SimpleEffort gate, but can be opened either with a wall-mounted button or a remote control. It also includes a motion sensor nightlight.
- SmartLight Stair Gate by Safety 1st
  Manufacturer Web site: *www.safety1st.com*

This gate is ideal for use at the top or bottom of stairs. For security at nighttime, this metal gate features a motion sensor night light that illuminates on approach. A secure lock indicator confirms when the gate is locked.

○ Safety Gate Installation Kit

● Safety Gate Installation Kit Model K10 for Kidco hardware-mounted gates
Manufacturer Web site: *www.kidco.com*
Kidco has assembled the materials and fasteners necessary to properly install any child safety gate to wood banisters, hollow wall, or wrought iron.

○ Extra-Wide Gates
These gates fit openings that are too wide for a standard-size gate.

● ConfigureGate Model G80 by Kidco
Manufacturer Web site: *www.kidco.com*
This gate is a unique solution for the odd-shaped space that does not have mounting points straight across. The ConfigureGate is the only build-your-own gate system. Wall-mounted for safety, it has three 24-inch interlocking sections that adjust in 10-degree increments and can be angled or set in a straight line as needed. Included in the three-piece basic set is a walk-through gate section that opens easily with a one-hand-applied adult release in either direction. The gate stands 29 inches tall.

The Configure Gate is a great gate if you want to block off part of a room just for the kids. The kids are still in view, and yet you don't have to worry about them getting into something that's dangerous.—Molly

● Élongate Model G60 by Kidco
Manufacturer Web site: *www.kidco.com*
This wall-mounted gate is designed to fit into wide, open spaces. It features a walk-through door that can be installed at either end. A simple, one-hand adult release allows the door to open in both directions. The gate expands from 45 inches to 60 inches wide. Optional 24-inch extensions will expand this gate up to 7, 9, 11, or even 13 feet wide. The gate stands 29½ inches tall.

- Expansion Swing Gate by Evenflo
  Manufacturer Web site: *www.evenflo.com*
  This wall-mounted, childproof, one-hand-release swing gate is convenient for high-traffic areas. Slam-latch locks are closed with a shove of the swing door. The gate expands from 24 inches to 60 inches wide and stands 32 inches tall.

○ Railing Guards and Netting
  Like many other parents, when you look at the banisters in your home, you probably think about your children's safety. If your deck or balcony railings have horizontal or vertical openings wider than four inches, you need to make some modifications. Railing guards protect your child from getting stuck between the rails or falling through. Railing guards also protect your pets and prevent children from throwing small objects through the rails.

  - Railnet by Safety 1st
    Manufacturer Web site: *www.safety1st.com*

We use the Railnet on our second-story deck. It keeps the little ones safe and allows us to relax while enjoying our time outside.—Tracy

  - Transparent Banister Guard by Banix
    Vendor Web sites *www.babycatalog.com; www.onestepahead.com*

PLAY-AREA SAFETY

Create a safe, enclosed play area in one room of your house. This area will provide all the space your children need, and you won't have to worry about them getting into things they shouldn't.

○ Play Den
  - PlayDen Model PD20 with Padded Floor by Kidco
    Manufacturer Web site: *www.kidco.com*
    Kidco's PlayDen is an enclosed, freestanding play area. The basic set includes six 24-inch interlocking sections that can connect and adjust to form many different layouts. When the PlayDen is fully set up, there's approximately 9.5 square feet of space inside. The PlayDen has a walk-through gate section that opens in either direction with a one-hand adult release. The 29½-inch-high vertical design discourages climbing, and it has a nontoxic finish, making the PlayDen easy to care for.

WINDOW SAFETY TIPS

Lots of windows are delightful in a home, but they can pose serious dangers for your little ones. Keep these safety tips in mind:

✔ Be sure that your home's windows, especially those that are several stories up, are secure, with sturdy guards.

✔ Ensure that any window your child has access to has some sort of mechanism that prevents it from opening more than 4 inches.

✔ Avoid positioning climbable furniture near windows.

✔ Do not put children's accessories such as highchairs, cribs, or playpens near windows or window blind cords. Use wind-ups (see below for wind-up recommendations) on any dangling cords.

✔ Remember that window screens keep bugs out, but they will not necessarily keep children in.

WINDOW SAFETY PRODUCTS

○ Cord Wind-Ups
A child can become entangled in blinds or curtain cords and strangle in a minute. Either cut cords off or use cord shorteners or wind-ups to keep them safely out of a child's reach.

● Blindwinder by Kidco
Manufacturer Web site: *www.kidco.com*

● Cord Wind-Up by Mommy's Helper
Vendor Web sites: *www.babyuniverse.com*; *www.safeandsecurebaby.com*

● Window Blind Cord Wind-Ups by Safety 1st
Manufacturer Web site: *www.safety1st.com*

○ Window Wedge
A window wedge controls the height or width of the window opening. Use window wedges on double-hung or sliding windows.

● Window Wedge by Kidco
Manufacturer Web site: *www.kidco.com*

What a wonderful safety feature. The Window Wedges are instantly adjustable so you can decide how high you want the window to open.—Janice

FIREPLACE SAFETY TIPS

Children are very curious when it comes to the fireplace. They love to climb up and down on the hearth, but taking a fall on the hard brick or marble can cause serious injury. Follow these tips to ensure fireplace safety:

✔ Cover raised hearths with a soft foam padding.

✔ Secure fireplace screens and glass doors.

✔ Secure all fireplace equipment.

✔ Keep firewood out of reach. Stacked firewood could tumble down onto your child.

FIREPLACE SAFETY PRODUCTS

○ Hearth Guards
Use hearth guards to prevent nasty falls onto hard fireplace surfaces. These falls occur too frequently to be ignored by safety-conscious parents.

● Cushiony Fireplace Guard by Prince Lionheart
Manufacturer Web site: *www.princelionheart.com*
The Fireplace Guard's cushiony foam absorbs impact and lessens the chance of falls causing serious injury to your child. Full-length double-stick tape keeps the Fireplace Guard securely fastened and removes quickly and easily when no longer needed.

● Fireplace Bumper Pad by Kid Kushion
Vendor Web sites: *www.babyage.com*; *www.babycatalog.com*
This bumper pad helps protect your child from serious injury by using thick pads made of safe, soft, durable foam. This product is flame retardant and non-toxic, as well as easy to install using the hook-and-loop tape stripes.

● Hearth Kushion by Kid Kushion
Vendor Web sites: *www.babyage.com*; *www.childsafetystore.com*
Securely attached around any fireplace, the Hearth Kushion is soft foam padding that protects your children from sharp edges.

○ Gas Valve Cover
If you have a gas fireplace, use a valve cover to prevent small children from turning on the gas valve. This cover will also keep dust and debris from falling into the starter keyhole.

● Fireplace Gas Valve Cover by Mommy's Helper
Vendor Web sites: *www.babyant.com*; *www.safeandsecurebaby.com*

OTHER SAFETY PRODUCTS

○ Small-Object Tester
If an object fits inside the tester, it's small enough to be a choking hazard. This item is a must for testing older siblings' toys when you have a baby at home.

- Choke Tester by Safety 1st
  Vendor Web sites: *www.perfectlysafe.com; www.safeandsecurebaby.com*
- Small Object Tester by Child Safety Products
  Vendor Web site: *www.safebeginnings.com*

○ Combination Smoke and Carbon Monoxide Alarm
Fire can break out anywhere at any time. Protect your family by having a smoke detector in every room. Carbon monoxide (CO) is the leading cause of accidental poisoning death in America, yet most people don't know they're suffering from CO poisoning until it's too late. Because symptoms of CO poisoning are like those of the flu, you might not even know you're in danger at first. That's why a CO alarm is an excellent way to protect your family. It can detect the CO you can't see, smell, or taste in the air.

Be sure to place a smoke and carbon monoxide alarm in every room in your house.—Janet

- Smoke and Carbon Monoxide Alarm by First Alert
  Manufacturer Web site: *www.firstalert.com*

○ Lead Testers
Lead poisoning can be deadly. If you live in an older house, be sure to check the paint and water for lead.
- Lead Test for Paint & Dust by Child Safety Products
  Vendor Web site: *www.safebeginnings.com*
- Lead in Water Test Kit by Child Safety Products
  Vendor Web site: *www.safebeginnings.com*

○ Fire Extinguishers
A fire extinguisher mounted within easy reach should be part of your home safety plan. If you can react to a fire when it starts, there's a good chance that, with the right type of extinguisher, you can stop the fire.
- Fire Extinguishers by First Alert
  Manufacturer Web site: *www.firstalert.com*

○ Fire Escape Ladder
If you live in an apartment or two-story house, a fire-escape ladder can give you an extra means of escape in a home fire.
- Fire Escape Ladder by First Alert
  Vendor Web site: *www.fireescapesystems.com*
- QuickEscape Emergency Escape Ladder by Bold Industries
  Manufacturer Web site: *www.boldindustries.com*

Chapter 9
Emergency Phone Numbers and Safety/Health Information

PARENTS' CONTACT INFORMATION

Parents' Names

_____

_____

Home Address

_____

_____

Home Phone

_____

Mom's Cell Phone

_____

Dad's Cell Phone

_____

Mom's Work Phone

_____

Dad's Work Phone

_____

Mom's Pager

_____

Dad's Pager

_____

MEDICAL AND EMERGENCY CONTACTS

Emergency Help: **Dial 911**

Pediatrician's Name, Address, and Phone

_____

_____

Poison Control Number

_____

Hospital Name, Address, and Phone

_____

_____

Hospital After-Hours Phone

_____

_____

Police Department Nonemergency Phone

_____

Fire Department Phone

_____

Gas and Electric Company Phone

_____

Taxi Service (Leave money in case of an emergency)

_____

Other Important Phone Numbers

_____

_____

HEALTH INSURANCE INFORMATION

Company

_____

Policy Holder's Name

_____

Group/Policy Number

_____

ID Number

_____

HEALTH AUTHORIZATION FORM

In case you or your contact person can't be found in an emergency, leave a healthcare form that authorizes your child-care provider to get medical attention for your child. If this form is not provided, your child may be refused treatment at an emergency room if a parent is not present.

FAMILY AND NEIGHBOR EMERGENCY CONTACTS

Local Grandparents' Names and Phone

_____

Relative's Name and Phone

_____

Friend's Name and Phone

_____

Neighbor's Name and Phone

_____

OTHER CONTACTS

Name and Phone

_____

Name and Phone

_____

Name and Phone

_____

Name and Phone

_____

Name and Phone

_____

Names and Dosages of Medications Taken Regularly

_____

_____

_____

_____

_____

_____

Medication Allergies

_____

_____

_____

_____

_____

Food Allergies

_____

_____

_____

_____

_____

Behavior or Habits to Be Aware Of

_____

_____

_____

_____

_____

Favorite Toys and Comfort Items

_____

_____

_____

_____

_____

Medications Are Kept

_____

_____

_____

_____

House Key Is Kept

_____

_____

_____

_____

First-Aid Supplies Are Kept

_____

_____

_____

_____

Flashlight Is Kept

_____

_____

_____

_____

In Case of Power Outage

_____

_____

_____

_____

Fire Extinguisher Is Kept

_____

_____

_____

_____

Water Shut-Off

_____

_____

_____

_____

Whenever you leave the house, be sure to let your child-care provider know:

- ✔ Where you will be
- ✔ Phone number where you can be reached
- ✔ Time you expect to return
- ✔ How to work the phone
- ✔ How to work the TV, VCR, DVD
- ✔ How to work the burglar alarm, if applicable
- ✔ Whether you are expecting visitors
- ✔ Any special instructions for that day

Having this sheet filled out, I can leave the house knowing my caregiver will have all the information she needs to know about my children and how to get in contact with the right person in an emergency.—Abby

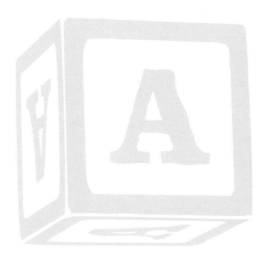

Chapter 10
Daily Feeding Schedule Sheet

Use this chart to keep track of baby's activities. Use it for a twenty-four-hour period (midnight to midnight), then start a new sheet. Only use the columns that apply to you. If you're not breastfeeding, ignore the four columns that pertain to pumping and breast milk.

Baby's Name: **Date:**

Feeding Time	Time/Amount You Pumped	Nursing Left (Min)	Nursing Right (Min)	Breast Milk from Bottle (oz)

When you're sleep deprived you can't remember anything. This sheet keeps me informed about what my baby has been doing. It's especially helpful if you have multiples.—Andy

Formula from Bottle (oz)	Pee	Poo	Comments

Part Two

Necessities and Nice-Things-to-Have Lists

Chapter 11

Newborn Necessities

Shopping for baby can be exhilarating, but it can also be overwhelming. There are so many products that it's hard to know where to start! Some store personnel will try to sell you anything and everything. So if you go in with some knowledge of what you need and how many of each item to buy, you'll be one step ahead of the game.

A newborn layette consists of clothing, receiving blankets, bedding, and other items you'll need when you bring baby home. Baby gear consists of the larger items, such as a bouncy seat, swing, and stroller. There are too many products on the market today to mention them all in this book. I've recommended the products I think are most useful, versatile, and the best buy for your money. This chapter lists the most popular brands and, in a series of parentheses, the recommended quantities of each item for a single baby, twins, and triplets, respectively. For example, at the end of the listing for prefolded or flat cloth diapers, you will find (4 doz.) (6 doz.) (8 doz.); this means that for a single baby, the recommended quantity is four dozen; for twins, six dozen; and for triplets, eight dozen. If a number isn't designated, purchase as many of the item as you feel are necessary.

You can find these items and brand names at most department stores, discount stores, and baby specialty shops, and on the Internet. (I've included manufacturers' Web sites and some vendor Web sites.) You can also refer to the Appendix, "Online Shopping for Baby," for a summary list of Web sites for baby items. Most manufacturers' Web sites will tell you where you can buy the product online or from a store in your area. You can look for a product at a designated Web site in one of two ways. Go to search, and type in the name of the product. If the product doesn't appear in the list, look for it under its brand name. If for some reason the product has been deleted from the designated Web site, simply go to *www.google.com*

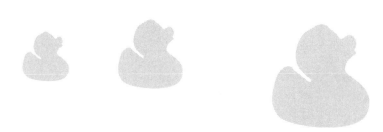

or *www.froogle.com*. Go to the search option on that Web site, type in the name of the product and the manufacturer, and the product should pop right up on your screen.

As in preceding chapters, you'll see a circle preceding each item or item category. Check off the item as you make your purchase. A streamlined, tear-out version of this checklist appears in Chapter 25: "Master Shopping List for a Single Baby, Twins, and Triplets." That list includes the name of each product, the quantity of each product you'll need to buy, and a space where you can jot down favorite brand names. You may not need or want to purchase every item listed below; select the products that you feel will be most helpful for you and your baby.

CLOTHING

Baby clothes are so cute! It can be a challenge not to overbuy. Remember, newborns grow fast—before you know it, your baby will be out of those first outfits.

FEATURES TO LOOK FOR

✔ Buy clothes that are bigger than your baby. Clothes shrink after they're washed. If they're a little bigger, your baby will be more comfortable and you'll get more use out of them.

✔ Cotton and other natural materials are preferable because they allow your baby's skin to breathe.

✔ If you choose patterns over solid colors, stains won't be as noticeable.

✔ When you buy socks or booties, make sure they are big enough so they won't make indentations on little feet and legs.

✔ Footed rompers and overalls with snap openings down the front and around the crotch are the most comfortable for baby, and they make changing diapers easy.

✔ Avoid clothing with buttons and ribbons. These items could pose a safety hazard.

✔ Buy a few of each item so you'll always have some ready to use while others are in the wash.

Once you've done your shopping and had your baby shower, wash all layette items and put them away before the baby is born. Then everything will be ready when baby arrives. And here's a little tip: If you receive clothing for baby in very large sizes, don't wash the outfit or take the price tag off. You might want to exchange it or take it back later on.

DIAPERS AND DIAPER ACCESSORIES

Figure that you will change your baby at least eight to ten times a day. You might be wondering, "Cloth or disposable diapers: which to use?" Some argue that using cloth diapers is environmentally friendlier. And if you wash them yourself, cloth diapers are much cheaper. However, you'll need to change baby more often if you use cloth diapers because they don't pull moisture away from baby's delicate skin. Sitting in a wet diaper, baby feels wet and cold—and may end up with diaper rash.

Disposable diapers are quick and easy to use. Because they pull moisture away from baby's skin, baby feels dryer and more comfortable throughout the day. Disposable diapers are also convenient because you don't have to bother with diaper covers, wraps, plastic pants, or pins.

CLOTH DIAPERS

Cloth diapers come in four styles: flat, prefolded, cloth with Velcro tabs, and all-in-one.

○ Prefolded or Flat Cloth Diapers (4 doz.) (6 doz.) (8 doz.)
Flat diapers are simple square or rectangular pieces of fabric, usually made of birdseye or gauze cotton, which you can fold to fit the size of the baby. Prefolded diapers have a thick layer sewn into the center of the diaper, which makes them more absorbent where absorbency is most needed. Both styles need to be pinned or clipped to stay in place, and both require a diaper cover or waterproof pants.

  ● Dundee Diapers
  Vendor Web sites: *www.bcfdirect.com*; *www.buybuybaby.com*

  ● Gerber Diapers
  Manufacturer Web site: *www.gerberchildrenswear.com*

- Kushies Diapers
  Manufacturer Web site: *www.kushies.com*
○ Cloth Diapers with Velcro Tabs (4 doz.) (6 doz.) (8 doz.)
  These diapers require no pins but still need a diaper cover or plastic pants to make them waterproof. The only drawback with Velcro tabs is that, after several washings, the Velcro tends to lose its stickiness.
    - Classic Diapers by Kushies
      Manufacturer Web site: *www.kushies.com*
    - Dappi Cloth Pinless Diaper by TL Care
      Vendor Web sites: *www.kidsurplus.com*; *www.tlcare.com*
○ All-in-One-Style Diapers (4 doz.) (6 doz.) (8 doz.)
  These diapers fasten with Velcro tabs and are convenient to use because the waterproof cover is attached, making diaper changing a one-step process.

The All-in-One style diaper is so easy to use. You don't need anything but the diaper. It already has Velcro tabs and a waterproof backing.—Jane

- Bumkins All in Ones Diapers
  Manufacturer Web site: *www.bumkins.com*
- Kushies Ultra (All In One) Diapers
  Manufacturer Web site: *www.kushies.com*
- Kushies Ultra (All In One Diapers) in preemie size
  Manufacturer Web site: *www.kushies.com*

DIAPER COVERS AND ACCESSORIES

○ Diaper Covers or Wraps (10) (12) (16)
  Most covers or wraps have Velcro tabs or snaps that fit securely and take the place of safety pins to hold a diaper in place.
  - Bummi Original
    Manufacturer Web site: *www.bummis.com*
    The Bummi Original has a superadjustable 3-inch tummy panel of Velcro that won't wear out. Soft and stretchy Lycra bindings provide comfort around the tummy and legs.
  - Bummi Super Whisper Wrap
    Manufacturer Web site: *www.bummis.com*
    Very adjustable, the Aplix closures have an innovative overlap design that ensures a custom fit on any baby. Durable, heavy-duty elastic

around legs and tummy will not wear out with repeated washing. Soft, smooth polyester knit bindings provide a comfortable, stretchy fit and a leakproof seal.

- Diaper Wraps by Kushies
  Manufacturer Web site: *www.kushies.com*
  These wraps are made of quality waterproof material and have easy on-and-off adjustable closures.

- EZ Cover Pinless Diaper Cover by Gerber
  Vendor Web site: *www.pottytrainingconcepts.com*
  EZ Covers are waterproof and have Velcro tab fasteners across the front. Elastic around the waist and legs prevents leaks.

○ Plastic Pants (8) (12) (18)
You can use plastic pants instead of diaper covers or wraps. Plastic pants can pull up over the diaper, or they might feature snaps on both sides.

- Dappi Vinyl Diaper Pants by TL Care
  Vendor Web sites: *www.tlcare.com*; *www.babybestbuy.com*. Click "Baby Diapering."

- Nylon Pull-On Diaper Covers by Tiny Tush
  Manufacturer Web site: *www.tinytush.com*

- Vinyl Pants by Gerber
  Vendor Web sites: *www.clothdiaper.com*; *www.kidsurplus.com*

- Whisper Pant by Bummis
  Manufacturer Web site: *www.bummis.com*

○ Diaper Pins (2 sets) (4 sets) (6 sets)
If you use diapers that require pins, make sure the pins are made of strong, rustproof stainless steel to ensure durability. Pins should have a safety-lock design that prevents unintentional openings while it ensures a secure, comfortable fit. To prevent accidental jabbing, always pin diapers going across baby's tummy rather than up and down.

- Diaper Pins by Sassy
  Manufacturer Web site: *www.sassybaby.com*
  Sassy diaper pins are made of stainless steel, which creates rustproof and sturdy pins to keep diapers snug on baby. For baby's safety, Sassy diaper pins are made with locking closures.

- Gerber Diaper Pins
  Vendor Web sites: *www.diapersite.com*; *www.tinytots.com*
  Gerber diaper pins come in three colors, with four pins per package— all blue, all yellow, all white, or an assortment.

- Metal Headed Diaper Pins by Dritz
  Vendor Web site: *www.clothdiaper.com*

These diaper pins have a safety locking feature to prevent the pins from opening when worn. They can be purchased in four different colors: blue, white, yellow, and pink.

- Plastic Headed Diaper Pins
  Vendor Web site: *www.clothdiaper.com*
  Plastic headed diaper pins work great for cloth diapering, baby shower invitations, laundry pins, and multiple other purposes.

DISPOSABLE DIAPERS

○ Disposable Preemie Diapers (6 pkgs.) (12 pkgs.) (16 pkgs.)

- Huggies Preemie Diapers
  Vendor Web sites: *www.drugstore.com; www.nurtureplace.com*

- Preemie Swaddlers Diapers by Pampers
  Vendor Web sites: *www.diapersite.com; www.kidsurplus.com*

○ Disposable Diapers (6 pkgs.) (12 pkgs.) (16 pkgs.)
Most moms like Pampers Swaddlers to start out with because they don't leak and they seem to be the most absorbent, especially for little boys.

- Huggies Newborn Gentle Care Diapers
  Manufacturer Web site: *www.huggies.com*

- Luvs Newborn Ultra Leakguards
  Manufacturer Web site: *www.luvs.com*

- Pampers Swaddlers Newborn Diapers
  Vendor Web sites: *www.amazon.com; www.drugstore.com*

NEWBORN LAYETTE

Before your baby's born, you'll want to be ready with a basic layette, and it's always good to have a variety of basic sizes and styles on hand to choose from, depending on baby's birth weight, how fast she grows, and the season of the year. The following list is fairly comprehensive, so you can choose what you think you'll need from the various categories.

○ Bodysuits or Onesies (5) (10) (12)
Bodysuits, or onesies as they are sometimes called, are one-piece undershirts that snap at the crotch to prevent the fabric from riding up around baby's chest and neck. When they're worn under a two-piece outfit, onesies help keep little tummies warm by keeping skin from being exposed.

- Bodysuits (a variety of brands)
  Vendor Web site: *www.babystyle.com*

- Bodysuits (a variety of brands)
  Vendor Web site: *www.babiesrus.com*

- Carter's Bodysuits
  Vendor Web sites: *www.jcpenney.com; www.macys.com*

- Gerber Onesies
  Manufacturer Web site: *www.gerberchildrenswear.com*
○ Gowns (5) (10) (12)
  For the first six weeks or so, babies live in gowns. One size fits all, and the longer the gown, the better; you can roll up the sleeves for newborns. Gowns are especially nice for nighttime wear because you don't have to fumble with snaps when you're changing your baby. Look for gowns that have a snap opening in the front, or no snaps at all.

Gowns are wonderful especially at night. They make diaper changing easy and there are no snaps to mess with.—Carolyn

- Gowns by Carter's
  Vendor Web sites: *www.babycenter.com; www.babiesrus.com*
- Gowns by Gerber
  Manufacturer Web site: *www.gerberchildrenswear.com*
- Infant Gowns (a variety of brands)
  Vendor Web site: *www.target.com*
○ Footed Rompers or Sleep 'N Plays (5) (10) (15)
  After baby gets too big to wear gowns, keep her warm and cozy in one-piece rompers or footed sleepers, and you won't have to worry about socks. Rompers and footed sleepers with snaps or a zipper up the front and between the legs are easiest to use. Rompers come in cotton, terry cloth, or velour. Plain terry-cloth rompers are most comfortable to sleep in, and printed rompers make cute everyday outfits.
  - Sleepers by Carter's
    Vendor Web site: *www.babycenter.com; www.jcpenney.com*
  - One Piece Playwear (a variety of brands)
    Vendor Web site: *www.babiesrus.com*
  - Gerber Sleep 'N Play
    Manufacturer Web site: *www.gerberchildrenswear.com*
  - Sleepers (a variety of brands)
    Vendor Web site: *www.target.com*
○ Sleep Sacks (2) (4) (6)
  Use a sleep sack when your little one outgrows receiving blankets and wiggles out from under loose crib blankets. Sleep sacks have a zipper from collar to foot, and a snap flap at the top for easy opening.
  - Back to Sleep Sack by Prince Lionheart
    Manufacturer Web site: *www.princelionheart.com*

- Beddiebye Plus Terry Wearable Safety Blanket by Kiddopotamus
  Manufacturer Web site: *www.kiddopotamus.com*
- Safety Blanket by Kushies
  Manufacturer Web site: *www.kushies.com*
- Sleepsack Wearable Blanket by Halo Innovations
  Manufacturer Web site: *www.haloinnovations.com*

*I sleep better at night knowing my baby is warm but
not caught up in her blanket.—Marie*

○ Blanket Sleepers (2) (4) (6)
  Use a blanket sleeper the same way you use a sleep sack.
  - Blanket Sleepers
    Vendor Web site: *www.amazon.com*
  - Blanket Sleepers by Gerber
    Manufacturer Web site: *www.gerberchildrenswear.com*
  - Blanket Sleepers by Carter's
    Vendor Web site: *www.babycenter.com*. Search "Blanket Sleeper."
○ Newborn Pairs of Booties or Socks (4) (8) (12)
  *Keep little footsies warm when baby wears an outfit without feet. Socks or
  booties should be snug enough to stay on, but not so tight that they cut off
  circulation or cause any indentation on baby's feet or legs.*
  - Baby Gap Booties and Socks
    Manufacturer Web site: *www.babygap.com*
  - Booties by Kushies
    Manufacturer Web site: *www.kushies.com*
  - Gerber Booties and Socks
    Manufacturer Web site: *www.gerberchildrenswear.com*
  - Newborn Socks by Zutano
    Manufacturer Web site: *www.zutano.com*
○ Sweaters (2) (4) (6)
  *Look for a sweater that has snaps or a zipper. If the sweater is a button-down
  style, make sure the buttons are sewn on securely and are large enough to
  button easily. You can find newborn sweaters at baby specialty shops and
  department stores.*
○ Newborn Hats (2) (4) (6)
  *Babies lose heat through their heads, so wearing a hat will keep them nice
  and warm. Make sure the hat fits properly—if it's too big, it could slip down
  over baby's eyes and nose.*

- Baby Cap by Kushies
  Manufacturer Web site: *www.kushies.com*
- Baby Gap Newborn Hats
  Manufacturer Web site: *www.babygap.com*
- Baby Jockey Hats
  Vendor Web site: *www.babiesrus.com*
- Gerber Caps
  Manufacturer Web site: *www.gerberchildrenswear.com*

○ Bibs (8) (12) (16)
Bibs protect clothing and keep baby dry when drooling starts as the result of teething. Buy bibs that snap, pull over the head, or close with Velcro in back. Bibs should have a waterproof backing to keep moisture away from baby.

- Baby Einstein Bibs
  Manufacturer Web site: *www.babyeinstein.com*
- Bibs (a variety of brands)
  Vendor Web site: *www.babiesrus.com*
- Carter's Bibs
  Vendor Web sites: *www.jcpenney.com*; *www.sears.com*
- Gerber Bibs
  Manufacturer Web site: *www.gerberchildrenswear.com*
- Hamco Bibs
  Vendor Web sites: *www.kidsurplus.com*; *www.netkidswear.com*

○ Receiving Blankets (6) (12) (15)
You can use receiving blankets for swaddling baby to make him feel safe and secure. Blankets come in thermal waffle weave, flannel, and cotton. Stretchy thermal blankets are the best for swaddling.

We love our thermal receiving blankets. When you swaddle baby he stays swaddled.—Melinda

- Receiving Blankets by Carter's
  Vendor Web sites: *www.babiesrus.com*; *www.babycenter.com*
- Receiving Blankets by Gerber
  Manufacturer Web site: *www.gerberchildrenswear.com*
- Receiving Blankets (a variety of brands)
  Vendor Web sites: *www.babiesrus.com*; *www.target.com*

○ Swaddling Blankets (6) (12) (15)
Swaddling blankets wrap like a receiving blanket. A preshaped pocket prevents baby from kicking off the swaddler.

- Easy-Wrap Swaddler by The First Years
  Manufacturer Web site: *www.thefirstyears.com*
- Swaddle Me Luxe Infant Wrap by Kiddopotamus
  Manufacturer Web site: *www.kiddopotamus.com*

○ Burp Cloths (2 doz.) (3 doz.) (3 doz.)
Use burp cloths to protect your clothing from drool or spit-up when you're burping your baby. You can buy specially made burp cloths or use flat-fold cloth diapers for the same purpose.
- Aware Burp Cloths
  Vendor Web sites: *www.babiesadvantage.com*; *www.greatbeginningsonline.com*
- Burp Cloth Sets
  Vendor Web site: *www.babystyle.com*
- Burp Pads by Kushies
  Manufacturer Web site: *www.kushies.com*
- Gerber Burp Cloths
  Manufacturer Web site: *www.gerberchildrenswear.com*

○ Lap Pads (9) (12) (12)
Lap pads are soft, felt-like waterproof pads that protect crib sheets, changing table covers, and any other surface you want to keep clean and dry.

They protect any surface from getting wet or dirty. We use them in the crib, on the changing table, sofa, anywhere we put baby down.—Cynthia

- Waterproof Lap Pads (a variety of brands)
  Vendor Web site: *www.kidsurplus.com*

○ Changing Table Pad Covers (2) (3) (3)
Keep your baby's changing table clean and comfy with a soft, fitted, terry-cloth changing table cover.
- Changing Pad Cover by ABC
  Vendor Web sites: *www.babyant.com*; *www.lullabylane.com*
- Contour Changing Pad Cover by Simmons
  Manufacturer Web site: *www.simmonsjp.com*
- Terry Changing Pad Cover by Rumble Tuff
  Vendor Web sites: *www.babycenter.com*; *www.lullabylane.com*
- Sleepi Changing Pad Terry Cover in Off-White by Stokke
  Vendor Web site: *www.babycatalog.com*

○ Hooded Bath Towels (2) (4) (6)
Hooded towels should be made of thick, absorbent terry-cloth material. The hood keeps baby's head warm after a bath.

- Carter's Hooded Towels
  Vendor Web site: *www.babycenter.com*
- Gerber Hooded Towels
  Manufacturer Web site: *www.gerberchildrenswear.com*
- Hooded Bath Towels (a variety of brands)
  Vendor Web sites: *www.target.com*; *www.babiesrus.com*

○ Washcloths (6) (12) (15)
Baby washcloths are smaller than standard-sized washcloths, which makes them easier to work with when you're washing your little one. Washcloths should be made of soft, absorbent terry cloth.

- Bumkins Washcloths
  Manufacturer Web site: *www.bumkins.com*
- Carter's Washcloths
  Vendor Web site: *www.jcpenney.com*
- Gerber Washcloths
  Manufacturer Web site: *www.gerberchildrenswear.com*

○ Preemie Clothing
Specially designed for preemies, these layette items are made of soft, 100 percent cotton.

- For the Love of Preemies
  Vendor Web sites: *www.babylinq.com*; *www.ittybittybundles.com*
- Preemie Collection by Gerber
  Manufacturer Web site: *www.gerberchildrenswear.com*
- Preemie Clothes and Newborn Baby Clothes Outlet Store
  Vendor Web site: *www.nurtureplace.com*
- The Preemie Store and More
  Vendor Web site: *www.preemiestore.com*

CRIB BEDDING

When you're shopping for baby's crib, you'll also need to buy a mattress and all the bedding to make the crib and mattress comfortable for baby. Bedding items include mattress pads, sheets, bumper pads, and blankets.

○ Crib Mattress—Foam or Coil (1) (2) (3)
Buy your mattress when you buy your crib. You'll have to decide between a foam mattress and a coil or innerspring mattress. Make sure the mattress is firm and fits snugly: There shouldn't be more than a finger's width between the mattress and all sides of the crib. Mattresses should measure 28 inches wide by 52 inches long, and they should be between 4 inches and

6 inches thick. They should feature a vinyl covering or other similar water-resistant material. If you're comparing high-density foam mattresses, pick the mattresses up. The heavier one is denser and likely better. The same criteria apply for coil mattresses.

We made sure we got a good firm mattress that fits snugly in the crib.—Allison

○ Foam Mattresses
Many parents prefer foam mattresses because they weigh less than inner-spring mattresses, and the lighter weight makes changing the crib sheet easier. Foam mattresses also cost less. The better foam mattresses are high density, about 1.5 pounds of foam per cubic foot. A high-density foam mattress should hold its shape as well as a coil mattress.

  ● Classica 1 by Colgate
  Vendor Web sites: *www.albeebaby.com; www.kidsurplus.com*
  This mattress is rated the number-one mattress by the leading consumer magazine. An extra-firm, orthopedic-style, nonallergenic foam mattress, the Classica 1 Crib Mattress is 5 inches thick and weighs only 7 pounds. The square corners hold crib sheets that have rounded corners.

  ● Visco Classica by Colgate
  Vendor Web sites: *www.albeebaby.com; www.kidsurplus.com*
  The Visco Classica is a dual-zone mattress. This mattress is used on the extra firm side for newborns and older babies. You can flip the mattress to the firm side for toddlers.

○ Coil Mattresses
Some parents prefer a coil mattress over a foam one because the coil mattress will keep its shape longer. Manufacturers equate the number of coils in an innerspring mattress with overall firmness, but that's not always the case. The wire gauge and tensile strength of the coils also contribute to the firmness, durability, and strength of the mattress. A coil mattress should have a minimum of 150 coils. An innerspring mattress should have coil rods that strengthen the innerspring mattress edge. Layers of cushioning material surround the innerspring to enhance support and provide surface softness.

  ● Sealy Baby Posturepedic Crown Jewel Crib Mattress by Kolcraft
  Vendor Web sites: *www.babycenter.com; www.livingincomfort.com*
  This mattress has all the benefits of a Sealy Posturepedic mattress scaled down to baby size. This 220-coil model ensures that the mattress will hold its shape, providing proper head and back support as long as you use it.

- Sealy Baby Soft Ultra Mattress by Kolcraft
  Vendor Web site: *www.babiesrus.com*
  Built on a foundation of 150 heavy-gauge interlocking coils, this standard-size mattress provides the ultimate softness and support for your baby.
- Sealy Tender Vibes Crib Mattress by Kolcraft
  Vendor Web sites: *www.livingincomfort.com*; *www.walmart.com*
  This mattress offers soothing vibrations to help your baby fall asleep. The 150-coil heavy-gauge steel innerspring unit provides maximum firmness. The mattress has an oversized on/off button for easy access.
- Super Maxipedic Mattress by Simmons
  Vendor Web site: *www.babiesrus.com*
  With 150 interlocking coils of 13.5-inch gauge-tempered steel, two firm fiber pads between coils, and foam polyurethane padding, this mattress offers the ultimate in back and spine support for your baby.

○ Fitted Waterproof or Quilted Mattress Pads (2) (4) (6)
A fitted mattress pad cushions the mattress and provides warmth so baby sleeps more comfortably. A mattress pad also protects the crib mattress from moisture. The pad should fit snugly around the mattress.

- Crib Waterproof Quilted Mattress Pad by ABC
  Vendor Web site: *www.babycenter.com*
- Ultrasoft Quilted Crib Mattress Pad by Continental Quilting
  Vendor Web site: *www.babiesrus.com*
- Waterproof Quilted Fitted Crib Mattress Pad by Continental Quilting
  Vendor Web sites: *www.babycatalog.com*; *www.kidsurplus.com*

○ Fitted Crib Sheets (2) (4) (6)
Crib sheets should fit tightly over the mattress so baby can't pull them off and become tangled in them. The sheets should be made of tight cotton fabric; flannel or knit crib sheets tend to fit loosely, posing more of a hazard to your child.

- Percale Crib Sheet by ABC
  Vendor Web sites: *www.babycenter.com*; *www.babyuniverse.com*
  Cotton percale crib sheets are available in a variety of colors to match your nursery theme.
- Carter's Crib Sheets
  Vendor Web sites: *www.babiesrus.com*; *www.jcpenney.com*
  Carter's crib sheets are 100 percent cotton, colorfast, machine washable, preshrunk, and extra soft for your infant's comfort. Crib sheet features deep pockets and reinforced corners for a premium fit.
- Crib Sheets (a variety of brands)
  Vendor Web site: *www.babiesrus.com*
- Crib Sheets (a variety of brands)
  Vendor Web site: *www.target.com*

- Gerber Crib Sheets
  Manufacturer Web site: *www.gerberchildrenswear.com*
  Gerber Crib Sheets are available in 100 percent ring-spun cotton or
  100 percent snug-fitting premium jersey knit. Deep corner pockets are
  tapered to stay on the crib mattress. Premium elastic helps hold the
  sheet in place. The tight fit helps prevent the sheet from pulling off.

○ Crib Blankets (2) (4) (6)
  Crib blankets keep baby nice and warm on cold nights. Crib blankets come in
  thermal, chenille, cotton, and fleecy materials. You can find crib blankets (a
  variety of brands) at baby specialty shops and department stores.

○ Bumper Pads (1) (2) (3)
  A crib bumper protects baby's head from hitting the crib slats. Bumper pads
  also keep young babies from sticking an arm or leg through the railings. Bum-
  per pads should fit securely in the crib with no overlapping, and no gaps at
  the ends. Avoid thick, fluffy bumper pads; the pads should be firm and flat.
  Bumper pads should have well-sewn ties at the top and the bottom, approxi-
  mately twelve to sixteen in all, with each tie between 7 inches and 9 inches
  long. When you insert the bumper in the crib, position the ties securely on the
  outside. Remove the bumper if your child likes to scoot under the bumper or
  press her face against it to sleep, or if she uses it as a step stool to climb out of
  the crib. Many parents coordinate crib bumpers with the rest of their crib bed-
  ding. If matching your crib bumper with the rest of your bedding isn't essential
  to you, you will find a good selection of bumpers at the following Web sites.

○ Special Bumper Pads

  - BreathableBaby Padded Mesh Crib Bumper by BreathableBaby
    Vendor Web site: *www.babiesrus.com*
    The BreathableBaby Bumper is a safer alternative to a traditional crib
    bumper. This two-piece, tieless system is easily installed and provides
    a secure fit. The bumper allows visibility and airflow for the child while
    she is sleeping in the crib. The white trim with white, slightly padded
    mesh will match virtually any nursery décor.

  - Crib Shield System by Trend Lab
    Vendor Web sites: *www.showeryourbaby.com*; *www.target.com*
    This pad set offers another breathable alternative to a traditional crib
    bumper. Consisting of four pieces that feature no ties but give a secure
    fit, it functions as both a rail cover and a side cover. Installation is easy,
    and you can remove the system for machine washing, or you can just
    wipe down the rail and side covers with a damp cloth.

  - Safe and Sound Bedding System by Cotton Tale Designs
    Manufacturer Web site: *www.cottontaledesigns.com*
    Cotton Tale Designs's crib sets consist of this Safe and Sound Bedding
    System: The four-sided crib bumper is totally enclosed on the bottom

and allows the mattress to fit inside the encasement, which eliminates the need for bottom ties and prevents baby from getting entangled or trapped between bumper and crib rails. This system is designed for a neat and fixed appearance.

○ Traditional Crib Bumpers
  ● Crib Bumpers (a variety of brands)
    Vendor Web sites: *www.babiesrus.com*; *www.babycenter.com*; *www.target.com*

○ Complete Crib Bedding Sets
  ● Crib Bedding Sets (a variety of brands)
    Vendor Web site: *www.target.com*
  ● Cotton Tale Designs Crib Bedding
    Manufacturer Web site: *www.cottontaledesigns.com*
    This is a quality bedding line of moderate price. They have two lines of infant bedding and related accessories available. These lines are called Cotton Tale Designs and N. Selby Designs. Both lines can be found in baby specialty stores and, as mentioned above, utilize the Safe and Sound Bedding System.
  ● Kids Line Crib Bedding
    Manufacturer Web site: *www.kidsline.com*
    From cozy nursery designs to innovative ideas for your child's bedroom, Kids Line products bring you the very best in design, quality, safety, and value. Each infant bedding collection from Kids Line promises a special space designed for the needs of your baby. Express your style with designs for boys, girls, or both!
  ● Lambs & Ivy Crib Bedding
    Manufacturer Web site: *www.lambsivy.com*
    Lambs & Ivy bedding sets can help create a nursery full of fantasy and wonder for babies. The bedding is available in many themes; you will find what you're looking for to create that special nursery.
  ● Laura Ashley
    Vendor Web sites: *www.babybeddingtown.com*; *www.dreamtimebaby.com*
    With Laura Ashley baby bedding, you bring style to your nursery. Laura Ashley crib bedding comes in adorable four-piece crib sets with Laura Ashley accessories to match.

BASSINET AND CRADLE BEDDING

Bassinet and cradle sheets should fit snugly over the mattress so they don't bunch up around baby. If the bassinet or cradle you buy does not come with a pad, you can find separate pads in various sizes at your local baby store or online. A mattress pad cover will make sleeping more comfortable for your baby and protect the mattress from moisture.

You might buy or borrow a bassinet or cradle without any bedding, but if you wish to dress up your bassinet or cradle, you can purchase complete bedding sets. Bassinet sets include a liner, hood, petite pillow, and blanket. Some sets come with matching sheets. Cradle sets include a comforter, bumper, and sheet. Have two sheets and mattress pad covers for each bassinet and cradle.

BASSINET BEDDING

- ○ Bassinet Pads (1) (2) (3)
  - ● Bassinet Pads by Colgate
    Vendor Web site: *www.babycatalog.com*. Search by brand.
  - ● Vinyl Bassinet Pad by Simmons
    Manufacturer Web site: *www.simmonsjp.com*
- ○ Bassinet Bumper
  - ● Bassinet Bumper by Baby Doll
    Vendor Web site: *www.ababy.com*
- ○ Bassinet Mattress Pad Covers (2) (4) (6)
  - ● Bassinet Waterproof Mattress Protector by Baby Doll
    Vendor Web sites: *www.jcpenney.com*; *www.ababy.com*
  - ● Waterproof Bassinet Pad by Carter's
    Vendor Web site: *www.babycenter.com*
  - ● Waterproof Bassinet Sheet by ABC
    Vendor Web site: *www.babycenter.com*
- ○ Bassinet Sheets (2) (4) (6)
  - ● Bassinet Sheet by Gerber
    Manufacturer Web site: *www.gerberchildrenswear.com*
  - ● Cotton Knit Bassinet Sheets by Carter's
    Vendor Web site: *www.jcpenney.com*
  - ● Jumbo Bassinet Sheets and Skirts by Badger Basket
    Manufacturer Web site: *www.badgerbasket.com*
  - ● Percale Bassinet Sheets by ABC
    Vendor Web sites: *www.babycenter.com*; *www.amazon.com*
- ○ Complete Bassinet Bedding Sets (1) (2) (3)
  - ● Bassinet Bedding (a variety of brands)
    Vendor Web site: *www.babyuniverse.com*
  - ● Bassinet Bedding by Badger Basket
    Manufacturer Web site: *www.badgerbasket.com*
  - ● Bassinet Bedding (a variety of brands)
    Vendor Web site: *www.ababy.com*

○ Cradle Pad (1) (2) (3)
- Cradle Pads by Colgate
  Vendor Web site: *www.babycatalog.com*. Search by brand.
- Vinyl Cradle Pad by Simmons
  Manufacturer Web site: *www.simmonsjp.com*

○ Cradle Mattress Pad Cover (2) (4) (6)
- Cradle and Bassinet Waterproof Quilted Mattress Pad by ABC
  Vendor Web site: *www.babycenter.com*

○ Cradle Bumpers (1) (2) (3)
- Cradle Bumper by ABC
  Vendor Web sites: *www.babycenter.com*; *www.lullabylane.com*
  Made of 100 percent cotton, these machine-washable bumpers are filled with 100 percent polyester batting.
- Cradle Bumper by Baby Doll
  Vendor Web site: *www.ababy.com*
  Beautiful pastel or primary colored bumpers are adorned with ruffles or tailored trim. These ultrasoft bumpers are filled with 100 percent cotton and are machine washable.
- Cradle Bumper by Koala Baby
  Vendor Web site: *www.babiesrus.com*
  This ultrasoft, 100 percent combed cotton bumper with polyester fill is machine washable and dryer safe.

○ Cradle Sheets (2) (4) (6)
- Cradle Sheets by Carter's
  Vendor Web sites: *www.babycenter.com*; *www.bcfdirect.com*
- Cradle Sheets by Gerber
  Manufacturer Web site: *www.gerberchildrenswear.com*
- Cradle Sheets by Koala Baby
  Vendor Web site: *www.babiesrus.com*
- Percale Cradle Sheet by ABC
  Vendor Web sites: *www.babycenter.com*; *www.babyuniverse.com*

○ Complete Cradle Bedding Sets (1) (2) (3)
- Cradle Bedding (a variety of brands)
  Vendor Web sites: *www.babiesrus.com*; *www.netkidswear.com*
- Cradle Bedding (a variety of brands)
  Vendor Web site: *www.ababy.com*

Sleeping with your baby for the first few months is an excellent bonding experience, but for peace of mind, you might want to purchase a product that will ensure you won't roll over on your baby, and that she won't be able to fall off or behind the bed. The following products will afford you that luxury. They can also be used as a crib insert and changing area, and they are ideal for C-section moms and all moms who must deal with nighttime feedings.

○ Baby Bed Inserts for Parents' Bed

- Close & Secure Sleeper by The First Years
  Manufacturer Web site: *www.thefirstyears.com*
  This insert features a three-sided bumper at the top, and a foot guard at the bottom. A patented airflow design allows air to circulate around baby, and a built-in night light makes it easy for you to check on baby during the night.

This product gives you the assured feeling that your infant is safe and sound right next to you in bed. You don't have to worry about rolling over on your baby, and nursing at night is a breeze.—Marilyn

- Deluxe Snuggle Nest by Baby Delight
  Manufacturer Web site: *www.babydelight.com*
  Snuggle Nest is recommended for use from birth to four months. Snuggle Nest comes with breathable mesh panels, a back and side sleep positioner, foam mattress, washable sheet, and cover. A clip-on minilight lets you check and soothe your baby without having to turn on harsh overhead lighting. You can find extra Snuggle Nest sheets at the same Web site.
- Deluxe Snuggle Nest Sheets by Baby Delight
  Manufacturer Web site: *www.babydelight.com*
  Extra sheets for your Snuggle Nest come in packages of two.
- Wee Sleep Bumper Bed by Leachco
  Manufacturer Web site: *www.leachco.com*
  This product is recommended for use from birth to six months. The Wee Sleep Bumper Bed includes bumpers around three sides and a padded mat for beneath baby. It's great for traveling with your baby, or for visiting relatives who do not have a crib available. The unit folds up for easy transport with its attached handle.

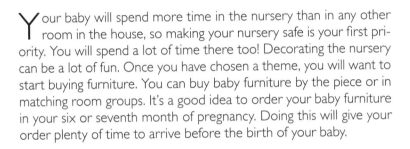

Chapter 12
Nursery Furniture

Your baby will spend more time in the nursery than in any other room in the house, so making your nursery safe is your first priority. You will spend a lot of time there too! Decorating the nursery can be a lot of fun. Once you have chosen a theme, you will want to start buying furniture. You can buy baby furniture by the piece or in matching room groups. It's a good idea to order your baby furniture in your six or seventh month of pregnancy. Doing this will give your order plenty of time to arrive before the birth of your baby.

CRIBS

A crib is one of the most important purchases you'll make for your nursery. The crib is the only place you will leave your child unattended. She will sleep in a crib until she's ready to move into a real bed, which most children do between the ages of two and three. So buy a crib that you will be happy using for the next few years. Also, never buy a used or antique crib. Older cribs might not conform to current safety standards and could jeopardize your baby's health. New cribs sold in the United States comply with modern safety standards. Look for a label that states the crib meets Consumer Product Safety Commission (CPSC) standards.

FEATURES TO LOOK FOR
- ✔ Slats should be no wider than 2⅜ inches apart, to ensure that your baby's body cannot slip through.
- ✔ Drop sides should be at least 9 inches above the mattress when the sides are lowered, and at least 26 inches above the mattress when the mattress is in its lowest position.

- ✔ The crib should have a railing that lowers so you can pick up your baby easily. Some cribs have railings that lower on both sides.
- ✔ Corner posts should protrude no further than $\frac{1}{16}$ inch above the end panels.
- ✔ Decorative knobs and posts present a hazard: They could entangle your child in her clothing.
- ✔ The mattress should fit snugly, with no more than two finger widths between the edge of the mattress and the crib side. A square-cornered mattress works best and is safest.
- ✔ Don't buy cribs with decorative cutouts that can trap a child's head or limbs.
- ✔ Buy a crib that's easy to move. Bigger, wider casters afford easier movement than small, narrow ones.
- ✔ The crib should have plastic teething rails.

CRIB SAFETY TIPS

- ✔ Follow assembly instructions carefully.
- ✔ For added security, use bumper pads for newborns and small babies. Be sure to remove bumper pads if your baby crawls under them, presses his face against them, or tries to climb on them.
- ✔ Keep railings up when baby is in the crib.
- ✔ If you move the crib, or change the height of the mattress, be sure all support hangers (the attachments that hold the mattress in place) are secure.
- ✔ Periodically tighten all nuts, bolts, and screws.
- ✔ Check plastic teething rails for cracks. Replace rails when sharp edges appear.

○ Cribs (1) (2) (3)

Cribs come in many different styles, colors, and wood finishes. There are stan-dard cribs, sleigh cribs, cribs with drawers, cribs with canopies, convertible cribs, and other models to choose from. The one you select for your baby will be based on your personal taste. When you are ready to buy a crib, start looking in stores or online to see what's available. Look at the various room settings. See which style and color best suits your home décor and price range. Following are some good Web sites for researching cribs and matching nursery furniture (search by "Cribs" at each Web site).

Manufacturer and Vendor Web sites: *www.ababy.com*; *www.babyuniverse .com*;*www.childcraftind.com*;*www.childrensfurniture.com*;*www.thenewparents guide.com*; *www.walmart.com*

CHANGING TABLE OR CHANGING-TABLE/DRESSER COMBINATIONS

A changing table provides a safe, convenient, sanitary place to change your baby. The amount of space you have and your personal style with regard to look and finish will determine which changing table is right for you. Chang-ing tables are available individually or in matching furniture collections to coordinate your nursery. Changing tables come in several different styles. Open-shelf changing tables usually come with a changing pad. Changing-table/dresser-drawer combinations, with or without a hutch, don't always come with a changing-table pad, so you might have to buy the pad separately. And make sure that you bolt the changing pad to the top of the dresser to keep the pad from slipping off while you're changing baby. If you don't want to invest in a changing table at all, check out the Rail Rider (see below for vendor information).

The following lists include a few changing tables in each style so you can get an idea of what they look like. For all styles of changing tables, search under "Changing Tables" at the listed Web sites. You will find many more options in the matching room furniture sections of the crib Web sites listed previously.

FEATURES TO LOOK FOR

✔ Sturdiness

✔ Comfortable height

✔ Changing table with a safety strap

✔ Large enough tabletop to accommodate a growing baby

✔ A protective guardrail

✔ A space where you can place diapers within easy reach

✔ A place where you can put diapering accessories out of baby's reach

○ Open-Shelf Changing Tables

The open-shelf style is your basic changing table. This style is convenient because everything you need to change your baby is within reach and in view. Listed are some Web sites where you can find examples of open-shelf changing tables.

Manufacturer and Vendor Web sites: *www.babystyle.com; www.netkidswear.com; www.thenewparentsguide.com; www.walmart.com*

○ Changing-Table/Dresser-Drawer Combinations

A changing table with dresser drawers lets you use the top of the dresser as a changing table and keep all of baby's diapers and clothing close at hand in the drawers. When your child outgrows the changing table, you can still use the dresser for storage space. Listed are Web sites where you can find examples of changing-table/dresser-drawer combinations.

Manufacturer and Vendor Web sites: *www.babystyle.com; www.jcpenney.com; www.thenewparentsguide.com; www.walmart.com*

○ Changing-Table/Dresser Combination with Hutch

This type of changing table offers the most storage space of all. It has both shelves and drawers, so you have lots of storage space right at your fingertips. You can use the shelves for diapers and diaper accessories, books, toys, or other things you want out in the open. You can use the drawers for clothing and other layette items. Listed are Web sites where you can find examples of changing-table/dresser combinations with hutches.

Manufacturer and Vendor Web sites: *www.ababy.com; www.poshtots.com; www.storkcraft.com; www.thenewparentsguide.com*

I can keep everything I need for our daughter right at my fingertips in the Changing-Table/Dresser Combination with Hutch. The drawers keep all her clothes within reach and the hutch provides extra space for her other necessities.—Pamala

○ Crib Rail Changing Station and Sheets

If baby's room is small, and you want to save space and money, check out the Rail Rider.

● Rail Rider by Burlington Baby

Vendor Web sites: *www.babycenter.com; www.babyuniverse.com*

The Rail Rider changing table creates a convenient diaper-changing surface right on baby's crib. It installs, without tools, on the rail of any standard crib and hangs out of the way when not in use.

- Rail Rider Sheet by Burlington Baby
  Vendor Web site: *www.babycenter.com*
  This is a soft, terry-cloth sheet for the Rail Rider changing table pad.

CHANGING-TABLE ACCESSORY

○ Changing-Table Pad
  Most changing tables come with a changing-table pad. If you are going to mount a changing-table pad on a dresser or other piece of furniture, make sure you measure before you buy the pad. Recommended pads come with mounting hardware for simple installation, or with a nonskid bottom surface to prevent the pad from moving.

- Changing Pad by Rumble Tuff
  Vendor Web sites: *www.babyage.com*; *www.babyuniverse.com*
- Contour Changing Pad by Simmons
  Vendor Web site: *www.babiesrus.com*
  Manufacturer Web site: *www.simmonsjp.com*
- Hi-Rise Three-Sided Contour Changing Pad by Colgate (Search under brand name)
  Vendor Web site: *www.babycatalog.com*

DRESSERS

If you have an open-shelf changing table and no other drawer space in baby's room, you will need some storage space for those cute little outfits baby will be getting. And depending on your needs and available space, you might want to consider a second dresser so you have a place for all of baby's clothing and accessories. A lot of expectant parents will buy a dresser that matches the rest of the nursery furniture, but any dresser will do. If you have a dresser around the house that you're not using, it will be fine for baby's room. If you are looking to buy a separate dresser, you'll find a wide variety to choose from.

FEATURES TO LOOK FOR

✔ Many dressers give you the option of drawer knobs or finger pulls. It's wise to select a dresser with finger pulls rather than drawer knobs because drawers with finger pulls are harder for baby to open. Once baby can open the drawers, he can use the open drawers as a step stool to climb up on the dresser.

✔ Dresser drawers that roll out on roller bearings will open more smoothly then drawers that sit on a track. **Dresser safety tip:** Anchor dresser to the wall, so if baby climbs, the dresser won't tip over.

○ Chests (1) (2)
The following Web sites show some very nice separate dressers (search under "Chests"):

Manufacturer and Vendor Web sites: *www.ababy.com*; *www.deltaenterprise .com*; *www.storkcraft.com*

OTHER USEFUL FURNITURE

In addition to all the basic baby furniture, many parents find several other pieces of furniture especially helpful as they care for their new baby or babies.

○ Glider Rocker
Gliders are perfect for the nursery or for any room in your home. The smooth forward-and-backward gliding motion requires almost no effort. Sit in the glider and bond with your baby, or just relax. A glider rocker is wonderful for feedings, and for rocking and soothing a fussy baby to sleep. Some gliders come with a multiposition lock. The multiposition lock mechanism enables the chair to be locked in place to stop gliding. This feature is especially useful when your baby falls asleep or if you do not want motion.

The Glider Rocker is a must for all nurseries. We don't know what we would do without it! It soothes our baby, helps him feed better, and fall asleep.—Mary

- Angel Line Glider Rocker
  Manufacturer Web site: *www.angelline.com*
  Angel Line offers well-constructed glider rockers in many different styles and colors to choose from.
- Dutailier Glider Rocker
  Manufacturer Web site: *www.dutailier.com*
  Dutailier's glider rocker provides the best solution to cuddle your baby in comfort. Rocking is comforting to a baby, and provides soothing relaxation. There are many different fabrics and finishes to choose from.
- Ultramotion Glide Rocker
  Vendor Web site: *www.target.com*
  The Ultramotion Glide Rocker comes with thick, comfortable cushions. Glide bearings offer smooth, soothing motion. Glider has soft edges and toxic-free finish. Cushions spot clean, frame wipes clean.

○ Ottoman
Designed to match your glider rocker, the ottoman lets you comfortably put your feet up while you're moving in sync with your glider.

- Angel Line Ottomans
  Manufacturer Web site: *www.angelline.com*
- Dutailier Ottomans
  Manufacturer Web site: *www.dutailier.com*

○ Small Table (1) or (2)
  A small table (or two, depending on your needs) by your glider or rocker will keep necessities within reach. You will be happy to have a place close at hand for baby's bottle and burp cloths, your breast-pumping equipment, a small clock, and other items. Any small table will do.

○ Arm's Reach Bedside Co-Sleeper
  The Arm's Reach Co-Sleeper lets you keep a single baby, twins, or triplets within arm's reach, without them actually being in bed with you, from the minute you bring them home. The Arm's Reach Co-Sleeper attaches to your bed under the mattress and is securely strapped into place. Whether you are bottle feeding or breastfeeding your baby, with the Arm's Reach Co-Sleeper you can reach over and draw your baby close to you without having to get out of bed. This feature is especially helpful if you've had a cesarean section. The Co-Sleeper is also convertible. You can use it as a changing table and a playard. The Co-Sleeper conveniently folds into its own nylon carrying bag for easy storage and travel.

What a wonderful invention! We have twins and wanted to keep them near us at night. They both sleep in the Bedside Co-Sleeper right next to our bed. I can reach over and tend to them all night without having to get out of bed.—Ashley

- Bedside Co-Sleepers by Arm's Reach
  Manufacturer Web site: *www.armsreach.com*

CO-SLEEPER ACCESSORIES

○ The following accessories are made especially for Arm's Reach Co-Sleepers.
- Arm's Reach Co-Sleeper Canopy
  Manufacturer Web site: *www.armsreach.com*
  The Arm's Reach Umbrella Canopy protects baby from the elements when she's outside. The cover fits Original, Mini, and Universal Arm's Reach Co-Sleeper Bassinets.

- Arm's Reach Co-Sleeper Fitted Sheets (2)
  Manufacturer Web site: *www.armsreach.com*
  Fitted sheets specifically designed for the Arm's Reach Co-Sleepers are available for all styles. The sheet assortment includes a 100 percent cotton white sheet, a 100 percent cotton unbleached natural sheet, and a cotton/polyester terry cloth (very soft) sheet.

- Arm's Reach Co-Sleeper Floor Length Liners
  Manufacturer Web site: *www.armsreach.com*
  Adorn your Co-Sleeper in a beautiful, quilted, floor-length liner created by Sweet Pea of California. Liners come in an array of colors to match any décor. The Deluxe Floor Length Liner fits all Original Co-Sleepers with the same snapping system and attachment means as the regular liner that comes with the base unit.

- Arm's Reach Co-Sleeper Leg Extensions
  Manufacturer Web site: *www.armsreach.com*
  The Original Co-Sleeper Leg Extensions raise the Co-Sleeper in 2-inch increments from 24 inches (normal bed height) to 30 inches (pillow-top bed height). When you use the full 6-inch extensions, you can comfortably use the Co-Sleeper as a changing table.

- Arm's Reach Co-Sleeper Netting
  Vendor Web site: *www.babycatalog.com*
  Co-Sleeper Netting easily slips over the Arm's Reach Co-Sleeper Bassinet Umbrella Canopy. Co-Sleeper Netting can only be used with your existing Co-Sleeper and Umbrella Canopy together.

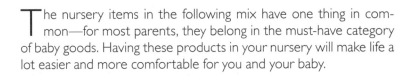

Chapter 13

Nursery Necessities

The nursery items in the following mix have one thing in common—for most parents, they belong in the must-have category of baby goods. Having these products in your nursery will make life a lot easier and more comfortable for you and your baby.

PACIFIERS

Pacifiers help satisfy a newborn's strong desire for sucking. Like bottle nipples, there are many pacifiers to choose from. For baby's safety, make sure all pacifiers you buy are a one-piece design. Pacifiers are sized by age range, from newborn to toddler. Latex pacifiers are softer and more flexible but don't last as long as the firmer silicone pacifiers, which hold their shape longer. Wash pacifiers often in hot soapy water, and rinse them well to keep them clean.

○ Pacifiers (3) (6) (9)
  - Avent Pacifiers
    Manufacturer Web site: *www.aventamerica.com*
    The Avent vented soothers can be steam sterilized, and each soother has a snap-on protective cap to keep it sterile until it's ready for use. Each pacifier has a safety handle, and they come in pairs in an attractive carrying case.
  - Binky Safe 'N Sure Pacifier by Playtex
    Manufacturer Web site: *www.playtexbaby.com*
    This pacifier features a nipple designed to simulate the shape of mother's breast to satisfy baby's sucking reflex.
  - Newborn Night Time Pacifier by Avent
    Manufacturer Web site: *www.aventamerica.com*
    Put an end to lost binkys during the night. The Night Time Pacifier's glow-in-the-dark handles make them easy to find.

- Nuk Pacifiers by Gerber
  Manufacturer Web site: *www.gerber.com*
  These pacifiers help baby's tongue, palate, and jaw develop naturally and simulate the motion of a mother's nipple while nursing.
- Soothie Pacifier by Children's Medical Ventures
  Manufacturer Web site: *www.childmed.com*
  Used in most hospital nurseries, the Soothie adheres to stringent American Academy of Pediatrics guidelines. The medical-grade silicone is the highest quality and latex free.

○ Preemie Pacifiers (3) (6) (9)

- Preemie Wee Soothie Pacifier by Children's Medical Ventures
  Vendor Web site: *www.preemie.com*
  Premature or small babies have a hard time fitting a regular-size pacifier in their mouths. These preemie pacifiers are just the right size for tiny babies.

DIAPER PAIL

Keep your baby's room or any room in the house smelling sweet and fresh by choosing a diaper pail that's easy to use and odor free. If you have a two-story house, keep a diaper pail upstairs, and a second one downstairs for convenience. You'll appreciate not having to run up and down the stairs every time you change a diaper.

○ Diaper Pail

- Diaper Champ by Baby Trend
  Manufacturer Web site: *www.babytrend.com*
  This is the best diaper pail on the market—no fuss, no smell, no special bags. Simply put the dirty diaper in the container on top of the pail and rotate the drum. The drum turns around, and the

dirty diaper falls into the pail. An empty container appears on top of the pail to start the process all over again. There's no need to lift lids or shove diapers into the pail. You can line the pail with standard garbage bags.

The Diaper Champ is so easy to use. Just drop the dirty diaper in, turn the handle, and the dirty diaper is gone! The Diaper Champ uses standard garbage bags so there are no special bags to mess with.—Jessica

- Diaper Dekor by Regal Lager
  Manufacturer Web site: *www.regallager.com*
  The second choice in diaper pails, the Diaper Dekor is a convenient, easy, and sanitary way to dispose of dirty diapers. It has hands-free operation; simply step on the pedal and discard the dirty diaper. You have to use Diaper Dekor with Diaper Dekor refill bags.

DIAPER WIPES WARMER

Warm diaper wipes make changing time more comfortable for your baby, and you'll be amazed at how much less crying there is during this time. Simply drop a stack of your favorite pop-up-type wipe refills into the warmer, pull a wipe through the small opening in the middle of the large lid, and you're ready for any type of diaper change.

○ Diaper Wipes Warmer
- Deluxe Wipe Warmer by Munchkin
  Manufacturer Web site: *www.munchkininc.com*
  This airtight wipes warmer has a refillable water reservoir and ventilation platform to keep moisture circulating around diaper wipes.
- The Ultimate Wipes Warmer and Ever-Fresh Replacement Pillows by Prince Lionheart
  Manufacturer Web site: *www.princelionheart.com*
  The Ultimate Wipes Warmer features the Ever-Fresh System. This system ensures that the warmer will never dry out the wipes. The Ever-Fresh pillow sits between the heat source and the wipes, helping to keep wipes moist and fresh.
- Wipe Warmer Ultra by Dex
  Manufacturer Web site: *www.dexproducts.com*
  The Wipe Warmer Ultra features a built-in changing light with auto shut off. The viewing window assures you that you will not unexpectedly run out of wipes.

SLEEP POSITIONERS

The American Board of Pediatrics states that babies should sleep on their back or side. These positions seem to be a positive factor in reducing the number of deaths caused by Sudden Infant Death Syndrome (SIDS). Sleep positioners hold babies comfortably on their sides or back in the crib. The safest sleep positioners have two short sides and no headpiece. (Never put anything around baby's head.) When you place baby in the positioner, never have the positioner come up higher than baby's shoulders. If baby starts to crawl out of the positioner, remove the positioner from the crib.

My daughter loves her sleep positioner. It gives her a safe and secure feeling, like being held.—Elizabeth

○ Sleep Positioner (1) (2) (3)
  - 2 in 1 Curved Sleep Positioner by Sassy
    Vendor Web sites: *www.albeebaby.com*; *www.baby-wise.com*
    The patented curved bumpers conform to baby's natural shape and accommodate both back- and side-sleeping positions.
  - Infant Sleep Positioner by Basic Comfort
    Manufacturer Web site: *www.basiccomfort.com*
    The Infant Sleep Positioner will help baby sleep safely on his back. This soft positioner has 45-degree dual wedges, with a machine-washable cover and removable foam.
  - Mother's Choice Sleep Positioner by Basic Comfort
    Manufacturer Web site: *www.basiccomfort.com*
    Mother's Choice Sleep Positioner offers excellent support, with 60-degree dual wedges. The Velcro-brand closure compatible mat helps to adjust the wedges for the perfect fit.
  - Proper Position or Proper Position Plus Vibrating Sleep Support by Leachco
    Manufacturer Web site: *www.leachco.com*
    The Proper Positioner keeps baby positioned on his back or side. The Proper Position Plus includes a push-button battery-operated vibrator guaranteed to calm even the fussiest babies!

BABY MONITORS

A monitor lets you listen to your baby any time of the day or night from any location in your house. A monitor consists of a transmitter and a receiver. Sounds can be transmitted as far as 150 to 400 feet away from the transmitter. Place the transmitter in the nursery within 10 feet of your child, and it will pick up the sounds your child makes. You can carry the receiver around with you or set it down in a specific place.

When you buy a baby monitor, look for specific features. The smaller the model, the more portable it is. Basic models have an on/off switch and volume control. The monitor should have a low-battery light that alerts you to the need for replacement batteries. A sound-activated light lets you glance at the monitor to see whether there is activity in the nursery. Double receivers give you the flexibility of keeping one receiver stationary and taking the other one with you as you move around the house or go outside.

How well a monitor works in your house will depend on where you live and any sources of interference in your home and neighborhood. If you live in the suburbs or country, a wide-bandwidth monitor will give you better clarity. If you live in the city, a low-bandwidth monitor will block out interference from portable phones, cell phones, and other monitors. Most monitors run on either household electricity or batteries. Some models act as an intercom or let you view your baby with a camera.

○ Baby Monitor

- Aquarium Monitor with Smart Response by Fisher Price
  Manufacturer Web site: *www.fisher-price.com*
  This monitor helps Mom and baby stay in touch with sound lights, crystal-clear reception, and a portable receiver. It also soothes and entertains with a ceiling light show, and soothing nature sounds. If baby wakes up, the Smart Response sound sensor actually "hears" baby's sounds and automatically responds with lights and music.

- Private Connection Monitor with Dual Receivers by Fisher Price
  Manufacturer Web site: *www.fisher-price.com*
  This monitor gives you a choice of ten channels to reduce the likelihood of someone picking up your transmission. And 900 MHz technology offers a more powerful signal, with excellent clarity and greater range than most other nursery monitors.

- Sounds 'N Lights Monitor with Dual Receivers by Fisher Price
  Manufacturer Web site: *www.fisher-price.com*
  The clear-view light display lets you not only hear but also actually see the different levels of your baby's activity.

- Ultra Clear Monitor with Dual Receivers by Graco
  Manufacturer Web site: *www.gracobaby.com*
  The Ultra Clear Monitor comes with two receivers so you can listen to your baby from more than one room at a time. Sound lights illuminate so that you can keep an eye on the sounds coming from baby's room.

○ Sounds and Movement Monitor

- Angelcare Movement Sensor with Sound Monitor and 2 Parents' Units
  by BebeSounds

Manufacturer Web site: *www.bebesounds.com*

Parents have a tendency to worry when baby sleeps. The Angelcare Movement Sensor with Sound Monitor is especially reassuring for parents with a premature baby or a baby with any type of respiratory problem. The monitor detects baby's slightest movements while she sleeps. If your baby goes absolutely still for twenty seconds, the sensor pad will send a signal to the nursery unit, which sounds an alarm that alerts you to check your baby. If you are out of the room, the two portable parents' units will pick up the alarm as well as other nursery sounds. The nursery unit has an optional "tic" feature. If the Sensor Pad senses movement, the nursery unit will continuously tick. If the pad doesn't sense movement, the ticking will stop. This "tic" feature is reassuring: If parents hear the ticking, they know everything is fine. The BebeSounds Movement Sensor will give you the peace of mind you won't get from a sound monitor or even a video monitor.

I was terrified that my baby would stop breathing and the only way I could get peace of mind was when she was sleeping with this monitor. I also loved the lights that lit up when she cried so I could peek at the parent unit to check on her. —Maggie

VIDEO MONITOR

If you're not comfortable unless you can see your baby at all times, then you will want to get a video monitor. A video monitor lets you keep your eyes, as well as your ears, on your little one.

○ Video Monitor

- Baby's Quiet Sounds Video Monitor Set by Summerinfant
  Manufacturer Web site: *www.summerinfant.com*
  This monitor has 900 MHz for superior clarity and range. The parents' audio unit comes with a belt clip. A night vision feature allows parents to see baby in a darkened room.

- Sight and Sound Assurance Video Monitor by Safety 1st
  Manufacturer Web site: *www.safety1st.com*
  This monitor includes a pivoting camera that allows parents to listen and watch their child on a 5-inch video monitor for complete reassurance. The portable audio receiver can operate on either battery power or electricity.

CLOTHES HAMPER

It's nice to keep baby's laundry separate. You can lift out the removable liner, with baby's dirty clothes inside, and carry everything to the laundry room. To keep liners fresh, wash them along with baby's clothes.

- ○ Hamper
  - A variety of hampers and styles are available for baby's nursery (search on "Hampers").
    Vendor Web sites: *www.babiesrus.com*; *www.babycenter.com*; *www.baby universe.com*
  - Badger Basket Hampers (a variety of shapes)
    Manufacturer Web site: *www.badgerbasket.com*

WASTEBASKET

Trash accumulates, and it's nice to have a place to put it.

- ○ Wastebasket
  - An assortment of cute wastebaskets to choose from (search on "Wastebaskets") follows.
    Vendor Web sites: *www.babybungalow.com*; *www.babyuniverse.com*; *www.badgerbasket.com*; *www.mercysake.com*

LAMP

Position the lamp so you can see what you're doing when you're changing baby without having the light shining directly in baby's eyes. Avoid a standing floor lamp because that can become hazardous when your baby starts to crawl.

- ○ Lamp
  - An assortment of nursery lamps to choose from follows (do a search on "Lamps").
    Vendor Web sites: *www.babiesrus.com*; *www.babyuniverse.com*; *www.kidsquartersonline.com*; *www.netkidswear.com*; *www.totsroom.com*

CLOCK

It's important to have a clock in the nursery, especially if you're breastfeeding.

- ○ Clock
    If you're looking for a special clock, check out the following Web sites (do a search on "Clocks").
  - Animal Wall Clocks by Tot Dots
    Manufacturer Web site: *www.totdots.com*
  - A range of clocks for baby's nursery
    Vendor Web sites: *www.babyuniverse.com*; *www.2blockheads.com*

- Cute Clocks by Platypus Productions
  Manufacturer Web site: *www.platypusproductions.com*

NIGHT LIGHTS

A soft, glowing night light is very reassuring to your child. A night light also makes it easier for you to find your way around when you get up for middle-of-the-night feedings, diaper changes, and pacifier searches. A night light will let you check on your baby without waking her up. Some night lights come with a portable flashlight in the event of a power outage.

○ Night Lights
  - A variety of nursery themed night lights are available on the following sites (do a search on "Night Lights").
    Vendor Web sites: *www.babiesrus.com*; *www.babyuniverse.com*; *www.switchhits.com*
  - Dim 'n Bright Auto Sensor Night Light by Safety 1st
    Manufacturer Web site: *www.safety1st.com*
  - Sleep-Tite Touch-Lite by Mommy's Helper
    Vendor Web sites: *www.babycatalog.com*; *www.kidsurplus.com*

HANGERS

Keep clothes neat and organized in baby's closet. You can find children's hangers at most baby specialty shops, and at drug and department stores.

○ Hangers
  - Children's Hangers, White
    Vendor Web site: *www.amazon.com*
  - Children's Hangers
    Vendor Web site: *www.thecontainerstore.com*
  - Children's Hangers
    Vendor Web site: *www.organize-everything.com*
  - Children's Hangers (a variety of brands)
    Vendor Web site: *www.netkidswear.com*

SMOKE AND CARBON MONOXIDE DETECTORS

A fire can break out at any time. Carbon monoxide is an odorless gas that can be very harmful, even fatal, if it's undetected. Protect your family by having a smoke and carbon monoxide detector in every room in the house.

○ Combination Smoke and Carbon Monoxide Detector
  - Kidde Combination Carbon Monoxide & Smoke Alarm by Kidde Safety
    Vendor Web site: *www.amazon.com*
  - Smoke Alarm and Carbon Monoxide Detector by First Alert
    Manufacturer Web site: *www.firstalert.com*

Chapter 14
Nursery Niceties

Plenty of products are not necessities—they're simply nice to have, if your budget permits. These products can make life a little easier or they can add a little something to your nursery.

BASSINETS, CRADLES, AND MOSES BASKETS

Many parents want to keep baby in their room for the first few months, so they think of a bassinet, cradle, or Moses basket as a place for baby to sleep alongside their bed. Bassinets, cradles, and Moses baskets are pretty and can be moved easily from room to room. The drawback to these options is that they are small, and baby will outgrow them quickly. Bassinets, cradles, and Moses baskets are expensive when you consider the short time you will be able to use them. To be more economical, borrow a bassinet, cradle, or Moses basket if you can. Some families have one of these items that they pass down from generation to generation. In the long run, if you're buying, a Pack 'n Play is more economical. If you still want the luxury of a new bassinet, cradle, or Moses basket, I offer some suggestions below.

BASSINET AND CRADLE SAFETY TIPS
- ✔ Never use a pillow for a mattress in a bassinet, cradle, or Moses basket. Pillows are too soft and can smother a baby.
- ✔ As soon as your baby begins to roll over and become more active, move him into a standard-sized crib.
- ✔ Make sure you follow the same safety guidelines for a bassinet or cradle as you would for a crib.
- ✔ If you use a Moses basket, do not carry your baby in the basket, and do not set the basket on anything but the floor while the baby is inside.

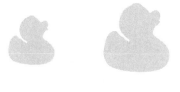

○ Bassinets (1) (2) (3)

- Bassinets (a variety of brands)
  Vendor Web sites: *www.ababy.com*; *www.ababysplace.com*; *www.thenewparentsguide.com*
  Complement any nursery with these beautiful bassinets, complete with bedding sets.

I loved the convenience of our bassinet. We could have the baby with us at all times by just moving it from room to room.—Justine

- Easy Reach Rocking Bassinet with Light Vibes by Kolcraft
  Manufacturer Web site: *www.kolcraft.com*
  This side-entry bassinet makes it easy for Mom to reach baby. The "Always There" Record-A-Voice soothes baby when Mom is away. A soothing vibrator and five classical lullaby songs help comfort baby to sleep. The bassinet has a soft-glow check light and soft toy mobile. This bassinet converts easily to a rocking bassinet.
- Tender Vibes Deluxe Bassinet with Music by Kolcraft
  Manufacturer Web site: *www.kolcraft.com*
  Tender Vibes has gentle vibration with variable speed control to soothe and calm baby. Five classical lullaby songs play to lull baby to sleep. Two soft toys hang from the canopy to entertain baby.

○ Cradles (1) (2) (3)

Cradles come in different styles, woods, and finishes. Check out the following Web sites to find the one that's right for you and your baby (do a search on "Cradles").

Vendor Web sites: *www.ababy.com*; *www.babyuniverse.com*; *www.thenew parentsguide.com*

○ Moses Baskets (1) (2) (3)

Moses baskets have removable mattress and bumpers, and the fabrics are machine washable. Carrying handles make it easy to transport the basket anywhere you want to go. As a safety precaution, never carry the baby in the basket. You will find beautiful Moses baskets, complete with bedding, at the following Web sites (do a search on "Moses baskets").

Vendor Web sites: *www.ababysplace.com*; *www.hoohobbers.com*; *www.the newparentsguide.com*

MOBILES

Newborns spend most of their time in a crib or bassinet. Babies need some stimulation during the day, and mobiles are their first form of entertainment. A mobile offers baby a close-up view of bright objects and friendly creatures that move to the sound of soothing music. A battery-operated mobile will run as long as you like; there's no winding every two minutes. When you get tired of the music, simply push a button or use a remote control to turn it off. Some mobiles even can be activated by your baby's own voice.

When you're choosing a mobile, get underneath the mobile and look at it from the baby's point of view. With many flat, two-dimensional mobiles, the objects seem to disappear when you look from the baby's angle. The best mobiles are three-dimensional, in which case the toys stand out. You should remove mobiles from a baby's crib when she reaches six months of age, or as soon as she begins to sit up. But removing the mobile doesn't mean you have to put it away. Many mobiles are designed so you can mount them on the wall for baby's enjoyment.

○ Battery-Operated Mobiles

  ● Colors & Shapes Musical Mobile by Baby Einstein

    Manufacturer Web site: *www.babyeinstein.com*

    The Colors & Shapes Musical Mobile with remote control plays classical Baby Einstein melodies and introduces babies to the sky, farm, and ocean. Hanging from this remote controlled mobile are colorful, plastic Baby Galileo, Baby MacDonald, and Baby Neptune characters, as well as various shapes with real-world sky, farm, and ocean-themed images tucked inside. Press the buttons below the baby-safe mirror and hear classical melodies from Beethoven, Brahms, Chopin, Debussy, and Tchaikovsky.

- Symphony-in-Motion Mobile with Remote Control by Tiny Love
  Manufacturer Web site: *www.tinylove.com*
  Studies show that listening to classical music can encourage certain types of intellectual and emotional development, a phenomenon called the Mozart effect. This unique mobile combines a multitude of fascinating movements and motions to captivate and stimulate baby's developing senses with the finest developmental classical music by Bach, Mozart, and Beethoven. This mobile has four different types of movement and motion. Beads slide from side to side as the arm turns and colorful animals or geometric shapes rotate as music plays. Three different songs play individually or consecutively for fifteen minutes. The mobile's arm is movable from side to side for convenience. The music box has a high/low volume adjustment. Symphony-in-Motion comes with remote control, so you can activate the mobile without disturbing baby.

- Symphony Light & Motion Mobile by Tiny Love
  Manufacturer Web site: *www.tinylove.com*
  This mobile is a celebration of music, nature sounds, and movement. It uses lights and liquid effects to stimulate a baby's development, filling her with a sense of calm and contentment.

○ Suction-Cup, Wall-Mounted Mobiles
A suction-cup, wall-mounted mobile can be hung anywhere in the house to entertain your baby. Hang it over the crib for play time; hang it over the changing table to distract baby while you're changing diapers. As your baby grows, you can hang the mobile in any room, out of reach, so baby can still enjoy it.

- Caterpillar Mobile by Sassy
  Vendor Web sites: *www.babiesrus.com*; *www.baby-wise.com*; *www.target.com*

- Zoomobile by Infantino
  Manufacturer Web site: *www.infantino.com*

○ Changing-Table Mobile
Keep baby entertained and happy while he's on the changing table with a mobile that clamps to most changing tables.

- Changing Table FlutterBug by Infantino
  Manufacturer Web site: *www.infantino.com*
  FlutterBug's spinning wings, bright patterns, colorful ribbons, and soothing tunes will entertain even the wiggliest baby.

- Jumpin' Jungle Changing Table Mobile by Learning Curve
  Vendor Web sites: *www.amazon.com*; *www.kidsurplus.com*

The lion, monkey, and giraffe move up and down as music plays "The Magic Flute." Each character has a special sound, and the characters can be adjusted to hang at various lengths to accommodate growing babies.

My baby doesn't like to lie still on the changing table. The Jumpin' Jungle mobile takes her mind off getting her diaper changed and being dressed.—Susan

DIAPER ACCESSORIES

Organize all of baby's changing needs! Make diaper changing quicker and more convenient by keeping diapers, wipes, ointments, and more right at your fingertips with a diaper and diaper wipes holder.

○ Diaper and Diaper Wipes Holder

- Diaper Depot by Prince Lionheart
  Manufacturer Web site: *www.princelionheart.com*
  The roomy bottom compartment holds sixteen to eighteen large cloth or disposable diapers. Baby wipes and a warmer sit on the flat tray, and the two removable side bins hold other baby necessities.

- Dresser Top Diaper Depot by Prince Lionheart
  Manufacturer Web site: *www.princelionheart.com*

○ Diaper Stacker
  You can use a diaper stacker to store diapers. Hang the stacker on the end of the changing table or crib—whichever is most convenient. Coordinate the diaper stacker with the rest of your nursery theme, or select a separate style.

- A variety of Web sites offering diaper stackers follow (do a search on "Diaper Stackers").
  Vendor Web sites: *www.babiesrus.com*; *www.babycenter.com*; *www.target .com*

ELEVATED SLEEP POSITIONER

Elevating your baby's head will make him feel better and get a better night's sleep. Pediatricians often recommend elevating the head of baby's crib to help baby breathe easier and sleep more comfortably after he eats. Elevating the head of your baby's crib helps prevent spitting up, especially for babies with reflux problems. This position is also medically helpful for babies with ear infections, colic, bronchitis, and asthma. Simply place an elevated sleep positioner under the sheet at the head of the crib.

An elevated sleep positioner helped my baby sleep more soundly, and he spit up less. It's great for babies with a reflux problem.—Ruth

○ Elevated Sleep Positioner (1) (2) (3)
  ● Folding Crib Wedge by Basic Comfort
    Manufacturer Web site: *www.basiccomfort.com*
  ● Safe Lift Crib Wedge by Dex
    Manufacturer Web site: *www.dexproducts.com*

NATURE SOUND, LULLABY, CASSETTE, AND CD PLAYERS

Even before birth, your baby can hear. After she's born, soothing sound machines calm her with sounds of nature, lullabies, or other relaxing music of your choice; and if she's fussy, she'll relax and drift off to sleep. If you have multiples, you might want one machine for each crib.

○ Nature Sounds and Lullaby Players
  ● Nature's Lullaby Player by The First Years
    Manufacturer Web site: *www.thefirstyears.com*
    Soothe baby by playing a choice of four preprogrammed audio selections, from comforting natural sounds to a medley of lullabies. The machine can be voice activated to go on automatically when baby cries, and then set either for shut off after fifteen minutes or for continuous play. This machine includes a soft, glowing night light.
  ● Sound Sleeper by Dex
    Manufacturer Web site: *www.dexproducts.com*
    This machine calms baby to sleep with a wide variety of nature sounds—there are more than thirty different combinations to choose from.
○ Cassette Player
  ● Crib CD Player with Night Light by The First Years
    Manufacturer Web site: *www.thefirstyears.com*
    Play your favorite music to baby anytime—soft lullabies to soothe baby to sleep or other musical selections to provide important audio stimulation when she's awake. The player can attach to the crib rail with a

child-resistant cover for safety. The player has a fifteen-minute timer and shut-off feature, plus a night light that you can turn on or off.

BABY SCALE

Many breastfeeding mothers are concerned about whether their babies are getting enough breast milk and gaining enough weight. Having a scale will help you keep track of baby's weight gain on your own. Knowing that your baby is gaining weight assures you that you are producing enough milk and your baby is nursing well.

○ Scale

- The BabyChecker by Medela—Weighs Infants and Toddlers
  Manufacturer Web site: *www.medela.com*
  The BabyChecker scale measures baby's weight up to 20 pounds, and toddlers' weight up to 40 pounds.
- The Baby Weigh Scale by Medela
  Manufacturer Web site: *www.medela.com*
  This scale measures the milk intake of premature and at-risk infants.
- Weigh to Grow Scale by WC Redmon
  Vendor Web sites: *www.babycatalog.com*; *www.babyuniverse.com*
  This scale converts to a normal scale as baby grows.

LAUNDRY PRODUCTS FOR BABY

Babies can and do get messy. Stains from formula, food, and the great outdoors can turn an adorable outfit into a garage-sale reject. But there are solutions to the stain dilemma. Here are several products that will keep baby's clothes smelling good and looking like new.

- Dreft Laundry Soap
  Available at your local grocery store or drugstore, this is a mild, sweet-smelling soap that gently cleans baby's laundry.
- Fabric Softener Dryer Sheets by Totally Toddler
  Manufacturer Web site: *www.totallytoddler.com*
  Unscented and dye free for sensitive skin. Use dryer sheets on clothing, bedding, blankets, stuffed animals, towels, and more.
- Nursery Fabric Softener by Totally Toddler
  Manufacturer Web site: *www.totallytoddler.com*
  This makes laundry fluffy soft. This product is made with a unique fragrance- and dye-free formula especially formulated for babies and children with sensitive skin. This gentle formula leaves clothes virtually residue free. It reduces static cling and wrinkles.
- Stain & Odor Remover by Mother's Little Miracle

Vendor Web sites: *www.pottytrainingconcepts*; *www.shopplanetkids.com*
These are nontoxic, natural liquid enzymes that completely break down organic stains and odors caused by spit-up, dirty diapers, food spills, and more.

- Stain & Odor Remover & Prewash by Totally Toddler
Manufacturer Web site: *www.totallytoddler.com*
This product is scientifically formulated to gently remove the most stubborn stains and odors.

- Stain Removing Wipes by Totally Toddler
Manufacturer Web site: *www.totallytoddler.com*
Now you can clean stains before they set in, which is especially convenient for travel stains. This product is the perfect size for every purse or diaper bag.

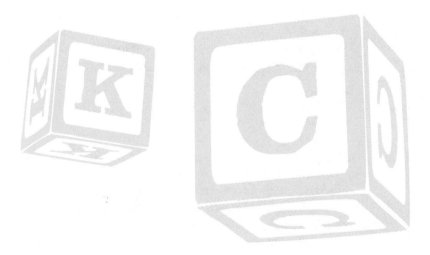

Chapter 15

Nursery Accessories

If you're looking for products to keep the nursery organized, smelling fresh, and looking cute, here are some suggestions. These accessories add color and charm to baby's room, and they help keep it neat, too!

○ Scented Drawer Liners
   Scented drawer liners keep your baby's nursery and drawers smelling sweet and fresh. Choose from several different fragrances. The coated paper has an easy-wipe surface, and the scent lasts up to two years.
   - Scented Drawer Liners by iPlay
     Vendor Web sites: *www.babycatalog.com*; *www.babysupermall.com*
   - Scented Drawer Liners by Lambs & Ivy
     Vendor Web sites: *www.babysupermall.com*; *www.dreamtimebaby.com*
   - Scented Drawer Liners by Taiusa
     Manufacturer Web site: *www.taiusa.com*

○ Closet Organizers
   With all the gifts baby receives, hand-me-downs from family and friends, and all the sales you couldn't resist, baby's closet soon becomes quite full of clothes in different sizes. Closet organizers make it simple to keep baby's closet neat and organized.
   - Baby Closet Organizer by Kolcraft
     Vendor Web sites: *www.babyage.com*; *www.walmart.com*
     This baby-closet organizer uses the space below baby's hanging clothes. Eight roomy shelves are perfect for folded clothes, diapers, and more. Six mesh pockets store socks, bibs, washcloths, and other baby accessories.

- Closet Cubby by Prince Lionheart
  Manufacturer Web site: *www.princelionheart.com*
  Teach your children to put away their things at a young age.
  Attach this great organizer to any closet rod for instant extra
  storage space.
- Closet Cubby Plus by Prince Lionheart
  Manufacturer Web site: *www.princelionheart.com*
  Double your closet space with this organizer. An extra hanging
  rod provides a place for those cute little outfits. Five roomy
  cubes hold clothes, shoes, toys, and more.
- Size It Closet Organizer—Newborn to Size 7 by Baby Buddy
  Manufacturer Web site: *www.babybuddy.com*
  These sized dividers make it simple to keep the whole wardrobe
  neat and orderly. Dividers range from newborn to size 7.

We got so many cute shower and baby gifts. I wanted my baby's closet organized by clothes size. Size It Closet Organizers come in Newborn to size 7 so everything could be organized accordingly.—Linda

○ Pictures and Wall Hangings
Use any pictures and wall hangings of your choice. Many parents like to match pictures and wall hangings to their nursery theme. You can find some really cute pictures and wall hangings at the following Web sites.
Manufacturer and Vendor Web sites: *www.kidsquartersonline.com; www.tots room.com*

○ Door Plaques by Platypus Productions
Personalize your baby's room with a door plaque with baby's name on it. These wooden door plaques are 5 inches by 8 inches and are available in many designs. The letters are all wood and hand painted.
Manufacturer Web site: *www.platypusproductions.com*

○ Growth Charts (I) (2) (3)
Children grow so fast, and little ones love to keep track of how tall they are getting. You and your child will have fun charting each new stage in the growing process.
- A Variety of Growth Charts
  Vendor Web site: *www.totsroom.com*
- Children's Growth Charts by Dolcemia
  Manufacturer Web site: *www.dolcemia.com*
- Children's Growth Charts by Watch Me Grow
  Manufacturer Web site: *www.watchmegrowup.com*
- Growth Charts (a variety of brands)
  Vendor Web site: *www.babyuniverse.com*
- Keepsake Growth Charts by Eeboo
  Manufacturer Web site: *www.eeboo.com*

○ Bookends
Baby will be receiving many books as gifts. Hold the books together on the shelf with a cute pair of bookends. Buy bookends separately or to match your nursery theme (when buying bookends on the Web, do a search on "Bookends").

With the emphasis placed on reading to your baby at an early age I knew we were going to get a lot of books as gifts. I didn't want them falling all over the shelf so I purchased a really cute set of bookends to hold them in place.—Jane

- Bookends (a variety of brands)
  Vendor Web sites: *www.babyuniverse.com*; *www.totsroom.com*
- Various Bookends by Platypus Productions
  Manufacturer Web site: *www.platypusproductions.com*

○ Children's Knobs and Drawer Pulls
  Create that special look in your child's room with adorable knobs and drawer pulls—there are so many to choose from. Coordinate your child's drawer pulls with your nursery theme. You will find a great selection of knobs and drawer pulls at the following Web sites. And keep in mind the safety precautions mentioned earlier regarding drawer knobs versus drawer pulls for younger children.

  Vendor Web sites: *www.babyultimate.com*; *www.kidsquartersonline.com*; *www .mercysake.com*

○ Switch Plates (a variety of brands)
  Cover up that plain light switch plate with a cute decorative one to match the décor of baby's room.

  Vendor Web sites: *www.switchhits.com*; *www.totsroom.com*

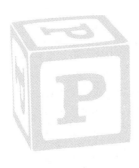

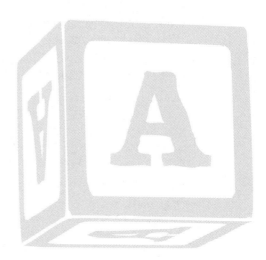

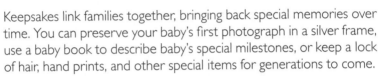

Chapter 16
Keepsakes

Keepsakes link families together, bringing back special memories over time. You can preserve your baby's first photograph in a silver frame, use a baby book to describe baby's special milestones, or keep a lock of hair, hand prints, and other special items for generations to come.

○ Handprint Sets
Little hands and feet don't last forever. Make beautiful plaster keepsakes of your baby's tiny hands and feet that will last a lifetime. Complete casting kits are safe, nontoxic, and nonallergenic.

  ● Handprint Kits by Child to Cherish
    Manufacturer Web site: *www.childtocherish.com*

  ● Ink Print Kit by Little Keepsakes
    Manufacturer Web site: *www.littlekeepsakes.com*

  ● Little Prints Tile Kit by 2000 Degrees
    Manufacturer Web site: *www.2000degrees.com*

○ Picture Frames
If you're looking for a picture frame to match baby's nursery theme, for baby's first sonogram photo, for daddy or grandma and grandpa, or one that's personalized or engraved, you will find a large selection at the following Web sites (do a search on "Picture Frames").
Vendor Web sites: *www.babiesrus.com*; *www.babyuniverse.com*

○ Piggy Banks
A piggy bank is a great addition to a baby's nursery. Teach your children the importance of saving money at an early age. Also, an adorable bank will make saving money fun.

  ● Big Belly Banks by Big Belly
    Manufacturer Web site: *www.bigbellybanks.com*
    Big Belly Banks are colorful, hand-crafted wooden characters with a patented coin track.

- Cute Banks (a variety of brands) (do a search on "Banks")
  Vendor Web sites: *www.babyuniverse.com*; *www.playtpus
  productions.com*
  You'll find an adorable selection of banks to enhance the
  décor of baby's nursery.
- Personalized Banks by Creations by Kim
  Manufacturer Web site: *www.creationsbykim.com*
  Hand-painted and personalized piggy banks make a wonderful gift. Choose from many different styles of adorable banks
  for kids of all ages. All banks come with a personalized name
  and design of your choice.

○ Keepsake Boxes
  *Keepsake boxes hold baby's first blanket, memory book, pair of
  shoes, and more. Built-in drawers organize mementos such as a lock
  of hair, pacifier, spoon, rattle, and other reminders of your child's early
  days. When your children are older, you will love looking back with
  them at some of the first things they called their own.*

*A keepsake box lets you collect all the special
mementoes of your baby's first year.—Cathy*

- Keepsake Boxes (a variety of brands)
  Vendor Web site: *www.babiesrus.com*
- Keepsake Boxes by Once Upon a Name
  Manufacturer Web site: *www.onceuponaname.com*

Chapter 17
Bath-Time Essentials

B ath time can be one of the most enjoyable moments of the day for you and your baby. Your new baby may initially resist the unfamiliar routine, but as she grows, splashing around with colorful bath toys will become good "clean" fun!

When you're getting ready to bathe your baby, make sure the room is warm and free of drafts. Fill the tub or sink and test the water for the proper temperature. Make sure the water is deep enough to cover your baby's lower body and tummy. Remember, babies like to be warm when they're taking a bath. Have all your supplies ready and nearby so you can dress your baby as soon as she is dry.

Some parents find a baby bathtub a waste of money, especially if they have a large kitchen sink. The kitchen sink is also a lot easier on your back. If you decide to use the kitchen sink, be sure to clean it with Lysol Antibacterial Kitchen Sink Cleaner before you bathe your baby.

The things you'll want to have handy at baby bath time are:

✔ Baby soap and shampoo
✔ Towel and washcloth
✔ Creams or lotions
✔ Diaper
✔ Onesie and outfit
✔ Receiving blanket

Here's a handy tip for bathing newborns. Wrap the baby in a receiving blanket before you put her in the bath. Doing this keeps her arms and legs from flailing about, and she feels safe and secure.

Slowly lower her into the bath, and gently unwrap the blanket in the water. Bath time should be a warm, happy, and fun experience.

BABY BATHTUBS

Safety and comfort are the primary factors to consider when you are giving your baby a bath. If you use a baby bathtub, choose a sturdy tub with a smooth, rounded edge that will retain its shape when you carry it full of water. Select a tub without a ramp. In a bathtub with a ramp, the water pools at the end of the tub, and your baby sits in the open air, wet and cold. As mentioned, babies like to be partially covered in warm water. Keeping warm is important to your baby's comfort and safety during the bath. Keep that in mind when you are choosing a bathtub. Because bathtubs with a ramp expose your baby to cold air, I've listed only bathtubs without a ramp. Some baby bathtubs have a heat sensor pad that lets you know if the water is too hot. But never rely on the pad alone; always test the water with your wrist or elbow before you place your baby in the tub. Many baby bathtubs have a drain plug and can be used in either a double or single kitchen sink, or in an adult bathtub.

❍ Baby Bathtubs
  ● Comfy Duck Bath Center by Safety 1st
    Manufacturer Web site: *www.safety1st.com*
    Ideal for infants from birth to six months, the Comfy Duck Bath Center features a comfortable and supportive tub with mesh sling. The bathtub has a supportive backrest with a slip-resistant pad and built-in accessory tray for bath-time essentials. A temperature strip helps ensure a comfortable water temperature for baby.

- EuroBath by Primo

  Manufacturer Web site: *www.primobaby.com*

  Bathing baby is easier and safer with Primo's EuroBath infant seat. It's the first "smart" bath because its unique anatomical shape keeps baby in the ideal bathing position and prevents him from slipping under the water. The extra-large 38-quart capacity and ability to place baby in two differet positions make Primo's EuroBath perfect for children from birth to twenty-four months.

- Sure Comfort Deluxe Newborn-to-Toddler Tub by The First Years

  Manufacturer Web site: *www.thefirstyears.com*

  The mesh sling with padded headrest provides extra comfort and support to cradle baby. Adjustable straps allow parents to change the height as baby grows. The deep, ergonomic design of the tub holds baby better for bathing. A special drain plug changes color to alert parents if the water is too hot.

- Tub-to-Seat Bath Complete by The First Years

  Vendor Web sites: *www.babiesrus.com*; *www.babyant.com*

  Tub-to-Seat Bath Complete will take you from baby's first sponge bath through graduating to the family bathtub. Use the bathtub in the sink or on the countertop for newborns and young infants. Store all of your baby's bathing supplies in the convenient drawer. When your baby can sit up, the tub easily coverts to a tub seat by using the storage drawer as a safety clamp that fits over the side of the family tub.

BATH SEAT

The most important thing when you are bathing your child is keeping her safe in the tub. Babies who can sit up on their own are ready for a bath seat, but do not rely on a bath seat for safety. Using a bath seat prevents your child from crawling around or standing up in the tub.

All bath seats should have suction cups securely fastened to the seat. All suction cups should securely adhere to the smooth surface of the bathtub. A straddle bar and safety belt on the bath seat keep your child from slipping into the water. **Bath safety tip:** Never leave your child alone or with a sibling in a tub of water.

○ Bath Seat

- Tubside Bath Seat by Safety 1st

  Manufacturer Web site: *www.safety1st.com*

  Washing your baby in the tub can be hard on your back. This bath seat does the swiveling for you, offering easy access to your baby's front, back, and sides while you stay in one comfortable position. This seat features an adjustable built-in restraint. Its "unique" arm locks onto the side of the tub to provide more stability for baby and a soft elbow rest for parents.

Our six-month-old loves to sit up and play with toys and splash her little feet. With the Tubside Bath Seat she never slips and I don't worry about her at all.—Jeanie

BATH-TIME CLEANSING PRODUCTS

When you are bathing your child, you will want to use only the best products for his tender skin. Look for mild, hypoallergenic formulas that won't irritate. Avoid heavily scented soaps and lotions, which can dry out delicate skin. Liquid soap lathers more quickly than bar soap. Also, liquid soap in a dispenser won't collect as much bacteria as soap that sits in a dish. And look for tear-free shampoos. If you find that a product irritates your baby's skin, try another brand.

- ○ Baby Bath Soaps
  - Baby Magic Gentle Baby Bath by Playtex
    Vendor Web site: *www.drugstore.com*
  - Essential Moisture Bath by Aveeno
    Manufacturer Web site: *www.aveeno.com*
  - Johnson's Baby Bath by Johnson & Johnson
    Manufacturer Web site: *www.johnsonsbaby.com*
- ○ All-in-One Body Wash and Shampoo
  Wash your baby from head to toe with one product.

I can wash my baby from the top of her head to the tip of her toes with one product.—Denise

- Baby Magic Gentle Hair & Body Wash by Playtex
  Vendor Web sites: *www.drugstore.com*; *www.medshopexpress.com*
- Baby Wash and Shampoo by Aveeno
  Manufacturer Web site: *www.aveeno.com*
- Grins & Giggles Baby Wash for Hair & Body by Gerber
  Vendor Web sites: *www.drugstore.com*; *www.walgreens.com*
- Johnson's Head-to-Toe Baby Wash by Johnson & Johnson
  Manufacturer Web site: *www.johnsonsbaby.com*

- 2-in-1 Hair and Body Wash by Mustela
  Manufacturer Web site: *www.mustelausa.com*

○ Vapor Bath Products
When your baby has a cold, you want to do everything you can to soothe and comfort her. The menthol vapors of a vapor bath provide soothing comfort for colds and sniffles.

- Grins & Giggles Vapor Bath by Gerber
  Manufacturer Web site: *www.gerber.com*
- Soothing Vapor Baby Bath by Johnson & Johnson
  Manufacturer Web site: *www.johnsonsbaby.com*

○ Shampoos
It's important to be careful when you clean baby's hair because her eyes are sensitive to irritants. You want to use the mildest of shampoos, and a shampoo that's tear free and hypoallergenic.

- Foam Shampoo for Newborns by Mustela
  Manufacturer Web site: *www.mustela.com*
- Johnson's Baby Shampoo by Johnson & Johnson
  Manufacturer Web site: *www.johnsonsbaby.com*

○ Cradle-Cap Shampoos
Cradle cap is a condition that causes baby's scalp to flake. This condition is characterized by a yellowish, scaly crust on baby's head that's caused by overactive sweat and oil glands in the scalp. Cradle cap isn't nice to look at, but it is not dangerous or contagious. Gentle treatment usually relieves this condition.

- Cradle Cap Treatment Products by Pure Baby
  Manufacturer Web site: *www.purebaby.com*
- Mustela Stelaker, for Cradle Cap
  Vendor Web site: *www.drugstore.com*
- Therapeutic Cradle Cap Shampoo by Little Forest
  Manufacturer Web site: *www.littleforest.com*

GROOMING PRODUCTS

Keep baby looking good, with hair neat and nails trimmed.

○ Brush and Comb Sets
Whether your baby has a lot or a little bit of hair, and whether it's straight or curly, thick or fine, a brush and comb make it easy to care for and style. Baby brushes have soft bristles that are gentle on baby's scalp. Baby combs have fine teeth with rounded tips for pull-free combing.

- Brush and Comb by Sassy
  Manufacturer Web site: *www.sassybaby.com*
- Comb & Brush by Gerber

Manufacturer Web site: *www.gerber.com*

- Comb & Brush Set by The First Years
Manufacturer Web site: *www.thefirstyears.com*

○ Baby Nail Scissors
The best time to trim nails is when baby is asleep. Baby is relaxed and not fighting to pull her little hands away. These child-sized scissors feature safety-rounded tips and easy-grip handles.

- Baby Safety Scissors by Gerber
Vendor Web site: *www.longs.com*

- Deluxe Baby Scissors by Safety 1st
Vendor Web site: *www.dmartstores.com*

- Soft Grip Scissors by Sassy
Manufacturer Web site: *www.sassybaby.com*

○ Baby Nail Clippers
Keep little nails smooth and neat. Many parents are afraid to cut little nails because they are hard to see. These nail clippers feature a magnifying lens that makes trimming a child's tiny, soft nails easier. Also listed is a standard baby nail clipper.

- Clear View Tweezers & Nail Clipper by Safety 1st
Manufacturer Web site: *www.safety1st.com*

- American Red Cross Deluxe Nail Clipper with Magnifier by The First Years
Manufacturer Web site: *www.thefirstyears.com*

- Fold-Up Nail Clipper by Safety 1st
Manufacturer Web site: *www.safety1st.com*

○ Emery Boards
If you don't feel comfortable cutting or clipping your baby's nails, you can file them with an emery board. Any brand will do.

○ Complete Manicure Set
Child-sized manicure sets include everything a parent needs to keep baby's nails smooth. Sets contain scissors, clippers, and emery boards.

- Three Piece Manicure Set by Safety 1st
Vendor Web site: *www.babyproofingplus.com*

○ Complete Grooming Sets
Good grooming habits start by having the right tools for the job. Get everything you need to keep your little one cuter than ever, all in one convenient set.

- 14-Piece Grooming Set by Safety 1st
Manufacturer Web site: *www.safety1st.com*
This baby-grooming kit keeps care accessories handy at home or on the go. A clear-view zippered carrying case gives each item its own

holder, plus plenty of room for extras. Kit includes a brush, comb, toothbrush, baby scissors, nail clippers, eight emery boards, and a sturdy travel case.

- Complete Grooming Kit by Safety 1st
  Manufacturer Web site: *www.safety1st.com*
  This grooming kit has all the necessities for safe and gentle grooming. Kit includes: soft-grip brush, comb, and toothbrush, baby scissors, fold-up nail clipper, four emery boards, and a zippered travel case.

○ Combination Grooming and Health-Care Kit
  These kits include both health-care and grooming essentials and feature all the must-have items a new parent needs.

- Baby's Deluxe Nursery Collection by Safety 1st
  Manufacturer Web site: *www.safety1st.com*
  Keep baby's grooming and health-care items organized at home or while traveling. The kit includes a digital thermometer with protective case, easy fill medicine syringe, easy fill medicine spoon, clear tip nasal aspirator, gentle care brush and comb, toddler toothbrush, steady grip nail clipper, baby scissors, tweezers, twelve emery boards, no scratch mittens, and a travel case.

- Deluxe Health & Grooming Kit by The First Years
  Manufacturer Web site: *www.thefirstyears.com*
  Keep everything you need to care for and groom your baby all in one convenient place. This set includes labeled holders for each grooming item, an infant brush and comb, sure-grip nail clippers and nail scissors, a fingertip toothbrush and toddler toothbrush, emery boards, a hospital-style nasal aspirator, a digital thermometer with case, a medicine dropper with travel case, a medicine spoon, a medicine dispenser, and a shake-and-see rattle. The zippered case has a storage pocket for extra items.

BATH-TIME ACCESSORIES

The following accessories will add comfort and ease to the bathing experience for both parents and baby. Again, pick and choose any or all of these items to suit to your needs and preferences.

○ Tub-Side Knee and Elbow Savers for Parents
  Enjoy greater comfort as you bathe your baby. Protect your knees and elbows while you're leaning over the tub at bath time.

- Sit & Store Tub Side Seat by The First Years
  Vendor Web sites: *www.babiesrus.com*; *www.onestepahead.com*
  Manufacturer Web site: *www.thefirstyears.com*

- Tubside Kneeler and Step Stool by Safety 1st
  Manufacturer Web site: *www.safety1st.com*

○ Spray Attachment for Bath or Sink

A spray attachment makes it easier to shampoo and rinse baby's hair without getting water in her face. The sprayer attaches easily to bath or sink faucets.

- Bath Shower Spray by Sassy
  Manufacturer Web site: *www.sassybaby.com*

○ Bath Visors

During bath time, visors help keep shampoo away from baby's face.

- Bath & Sun Visors by Sassy
  Manufacturer Web site: *www.sassybaby.com*

- Sudsy Sun Shield Shampoo and Sun Visor by Kel-Gar
  Manufacturer Web site: *www.kelgar.com*

○ Toy Bags and Organizers

Keep the bathroom tidy by storing bath toys in a toy bag. Toy bags use easy-to-install and quick-to-remove suction cups that mount securely to any smooth surface.

- Bath Toy Bag by Safety 1st
  Manufacturer Web site: *www.safety1st.com*

- Large Tub Toy Organizer by Sassy
  Manufacturer Web site: *www.sassybaby.com*

- Multi-Purpose Toy Hammock by Prince Lionheart
  Manufacturer Web site: *www.princelionheart.com*

- Sudsy Storage Tub Toy Holder/Organizer by Kel-Gar
  Manufacturer Web site: *www.kelgar.com*

- Tub Toy Organizer by Sassy
  Manufacturer Web site: *www.sassybaby.com*

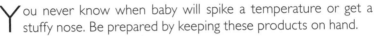

Chapter 18

Health-Care Products

You never know when baby will spike a temperature or get a stuffy nose. Be prepared by keeping these products on hand.

○ Digital Thermometer (1) (2) (2)
Glass thermometers are no longer recommended because of the mercury they contain. The most commonly used thermometers are digital; you can use most of them orally, under the arm, or rectally.

- 10-Second Thermometer by The First Years
  Manufacturer Web site: *www.thefirstyears.com*

- 8-Second Thermometer by Safety 1st
  Manufacturer Web site: *www.safety1st.com*

- Swift Read 3-in-1 Thermometer by Safety 1st
  Manufacturer Web site: *www.safety1st.com*

○ Nasal Aspirator (1) (2) (3)
A nasal aspirator is used to suction out nasal congestion. You can use an aspirator with or without administering infant saline nose drops. First make sure the tip of the aspirator is small enough to fit in baby's nose. Before you insert the aspirator tip into baby's nostril, squeeze the bulb to allow the air to escape. Then gently insert the tip into baby's nostril, and slowly release the bulb to allow suction to draw mucous from the nasal passage. To clean the bulb, squeeze to empty the contents, and then wash with warm soapy water inside and out, and rinse well.

- American Red Cross Hospital-Style Nasal Aspirator by The First Years
  Manufacturer Web site: *www.thefirstyears.com*

- Nasal Aspirator by Safety 1st
  Manufacturer Web site: *www.safety1st.com*

- Preemie Nasal Aspirator by Safety 1st
  Manufacturer Web site: *www.safety1st.com*

○ Infant Saline Nose Drops
Saline nose drops for infants help clear congestion from stuffy little noses. Infant saline nose drops are not medicated. Administer a few drops in each nostril, and then suction out with a nasal aspirator.

When our baby came down with a cold, the only thing that would clear her nose was administering some infant saline nose drops and sucking them out with a nasal aspirator.—Pat

- Ayr Baby Saline Nose Spray/Drops for Infants and Children
  Vendor Web sites: *www.drugstore.com; www.walgreens.com*
- Saline Spray/Drops by Little Noses
  Vendor Web sites: *www.drugstore.com; www.walgreens.com*

○ Cotton Swabs
You will use cotton swabs with rubbing alcohol to clean the base of the umbilical cord. Doing this promotes faster healing.
- Cotton Swabs by Q-tips
  Vendor Web sites: *www.drugstore.com; www.walgreens.com*
- Cotton Swabs by Johnson & Johnson
  Vendor Web sites: *www.drugstore.com; www.longs.com*

○ Rubbing Alcohol
Used to care for baby's umbilical cord and to clean the thermometer.
- Rubbing Alcohol
  Vendor Web sites: *www.drugstore.com; www.longs.com*

○ Small Jar of Petroleum Jelly and 2" by 2" Sterile Gauze Pads
You will use Vaseline to protect baby's bottom from diaper rash, to lubricate the tip of a thermometer when you're taking your baby's temperature rectally, and to care for baby's circumcision site. If you have a boy who has been circumcised, put a little Vaseline on a 2 inch by 2 inch sterile gauze pad and place the pad over the circumcision site. Doing this will help heal the circumcision and keep the diaper from sticking to the circumcised area.

- Vaseline—Nursery Jelly Baby Fresh Scent
  Vendor Web sites: *www.drugstore.com*; *www.walgreens.com*

○ Calibrated Medication Dispenser
You'll use a medicine dispenser to measure and administer medications.

- The Medicator by Munchkin
  Manufacturer Web site: *www.munchkininc.com*
- Medicine Dropper by Safety 1st
  Manufacturer Web site: *www.safety1st.com*
- Soft Tip Medicine Dispenser by The First Years
  Manufacturer Web site: *www.thefirstyears.com*

○ Fever Reducer
A fever reducer relieves pain and reduces fever caused by illness, teething, or immunization reactions.

- Tylenol Infant Drops
  Vendor Web sites: *www.drugstore.com*; *www.walgreens.com*

○ Gas-Relief Drops
Gas-relief drops relieve baby's pain and cramping from gas. You do not need a prescription for gas-relief drops; you can buy them over the counter in drugstores or pharmacies. You can give the drops frequently throughout the day—and they really do work. You can find all gas-drops products at *www.colicshop .com* in addition to the other listed Web sites.

- Gas Relief Drops by Gerber
  Vendor Web sites: *www.colicshop.com*; *www.thebabyoutlet.com*
- Gas Relief Drops—Natural Berry Flavor by Little Tummys
  Vendor Web sites: *www.drugstore.com*; *www.walgreens.com*
- Gripe Water by Baby Bliss
  Manufacturer Web site: *www.baby-bliss.com*
- Infant Mylicon Drops by Johnson & Johnson
  Vendor Web sites: *www.drugstore.com*; *www.walgreens.com*

○ Infant Glycerin Suppositories
Infant glycerin suppositories are for the relief of temporary constipation. You should consult your pediatrician before you use them.

- Glycerin Suppositories—Infant Laxative by Longs Drugs
  Manufacturer Web site: *www.longs.com*

○ Teething Gel
Teething gel relieves the pain of sore, swollen gums caused by teething.
- Baby Anbesol by Anbesol
  Manufacturer Web site: *www.anbesol.com*
- Baby Orajel Nighttime Formula by Orajel
  Manufacturer Web site: *www.orajel.com*
- Baby Orajel Teething Pain Swabs by Orajel
  Manufacturer Web site: *www.orajel.com*
- Oral Pain Relief Gel by Little Remedies
  Manufacturer Web site: *www.littleremedies.com*

○ Vaporizer
A vaporizer helps break up congestion when your child has a respiratory illness.
- Vicks Vaporizer with Night Light by Vicks
  Vendor Web sites: *www.drugstore.com*; *www.medshopexpress.com*
- Waterless Vaporizer by Evenflo
  Vendor Web sites: *www.amazon.com*; *www.babyage.com*

○ Humidifier
If a baby's nose seems stuffy all the time, the condition might be to the result of dry, warm air. A humidifier will add moisture to the air and help relieve congestion.
- American Red Cross Cool Mist Humidifier by The First Years
  Manufacturer Web site: *www.thefirstyears.com*
- Cool Mist Humidifier by Vicks
  Vendor Web sites: *www.drugstore.com*; *www.walgreens.com*
- Cool Mist Humidifier by Walgreens
  Vendor Web site: *www.walgreens.com*

○ Health-Care Kits
Health-care kits are perfect for first-time parents. These kits contain many of the basic health-care items in one convenient package.
- American Red Cross Deluxe Health Care Kit by The First Years
  Manufacturer Web site: *www.thefirstyears.com*
  The Deluxe Health Care Kit includes comfort-care nail clippers, a comfort-care medicine spoon, a soft tip medicine dispenser, a comfort-care nasal aspirator, and a baby digital thermometer with case. All these items fit into a handy carrying case that has labeled holders to keep everything in its place. A handy grooming and wellness guide includes helpful tips and complete usage instructions.
- 6-Piece Nursery Care Kit by Safety 1st
  Manufacturer Web site: *www.safety1st.com*
  This kit includes a digital thermometer, medicine dropper, nasal aspirator, medicine spoon, nail clipper, and reusable drawer organizer.

Chapter 19
Skin-Care Products

Diaper rash and the elements can irritate baby's delicate skin. Diaper-rash creams, soothing lotions, and sunscreen products protect baby's skin and keep it rash free, soft, and healthy. In addition to the listed Web sites, you can find these products in your local drugstores, grocery stores, and baby specialty shops.

○ Non-Allergenic Diaper Wipes
Diaper wipes are the easy way to clean up after messy diapers. Alcohol free and hypoallergenic, scented or fragrance free, diaper wipes provide gentle, skin-soothing cleansing while they moisturize baby's delicate skin. Select a thick, strong, quilted wipe so your fingers won't poke through when you remove the wipes from the container. Wipes come in their own original containers or in refill packs. If you are going to use a diaper-wipes warmer, the refill packs are more convenient. The following are popular brands.

[Diaper wipes] are gentle on my baby's bottom and keep her diaper-rash free.—Bobbie

- Cleansing and Soothing Wipes for Diaper Change by Mustela
  Manufacturer Web site: *www.mustelausa.com*
- Huggies and Pampers Wipes
  Vendor Web sites: *www.drugstore.com*; *www.longs.com*
- Luvs Diaper Wipes
  Manufacturer Web site: *www.luvs.com*

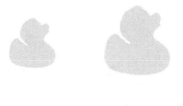

- Tushies Diaper Wipes
  Manufacturer Web site: *www.tushies.com*

○ Diaper-Rash Creams and Ointments
Diaper-rash ointment helps prevent or treat diaper rash. Diaper-rash ointments and creams contain zinc oxide, the ingredient pediatricians recommend to provide the extra care your baby's tender skin needs when he has diaper rash. The following are popular brands of diaper-rash creams and ointments.

- Balmex, Desitin, Desitin Creamy
  Vendor Web site: *www.drugstore.com*
- Boudreaux's Butt Paste, Desitin, Desitin Creamy
  Vendor Web site: *www.walgreens.com*
- Calendula Baby Cream by Weleda
  Vendor Web site: *www.drugstore.com*
- Calendula Cream by California Baby
  Manufacturer Web site: *www.californiababy.com*

○ Baby Lotions
Baby lotion will moisturize and soothe your baby's skin and protect it from drying and cracking. Use baby lotion any time baby has dry skin.

My newborn had very dry, cracked, flaky skin. By applying baby lotion twice a day her skin was soft and smooth in a few days.—Amy

- Baby Magic Lotion by Playtex
  Vendor Web sites: *www.americarx.com*; *www.familymeds.com*
- Daily Moisture Lotion by Aveeno
  Manufacturer Web site: *www.aveeno.com*
- Gerber Baby Lotion by Gerber
  Vendor Web sites: *www.americarx.com*; *www.drugstore.com*
- Hydra-Bebe Body Lotion by Mustela
  Manufacturer Web site: *www.mustela.com*
- Johnson's Baby Lotion by Johnson & Johnson
  Manufacturer Web site: *www.johnsonsbaby.com*

○ Sunscreen Lotions and Sprays
  Sun block protects baby from UVB and UVA rays. You should not use sunscreen on babies under six months of age.
- Coppertone Water BABIES Spectra3 Sunblock Lotion—SPF 50 by Coppertone
  Manufacturer Web site: *www.coppertone.com*
- Everyday/Year-Round SPF 30+ Sunscreen Lotion by California Baby
  Manufacturer Web site: *www.californiababy.com*
- Very High Sun Protection Lotion—SPF 50 by Mustela
  Manufacturer Web site: *www.mustela.com*

I love to take my baby for long walks, especially in the summertime, but I worry about the effect of the sun on her skin. Knowing I have these wonderful sunscreen lotions and sprays to protect her delicate skin alleviates my fear of her being exposed to the sun.—Kim

○ Sun-Block Stick
  With sun block in stick form, you don't need to worry so much about getting it in your children's eyes. Sun-block stick is great to touch up sun-sensitive areas such as lips, noses, and cheeks.
- Coppertone Water BABIES Sunblock Stick—SPF 30 by Coppertone
  Manufacturer Web site: *www.coppertone.com*

- Everyday/Year-Round SPF 30+ Sunblock Stick by California Baby
  Manufacturer Web site: *www.californiababy.com*

○ Soothing Products for Dry or Sunburned Skin
  After a day in the sun, these lotions and sprays gently hydrate and soothe dry or sunburned skin.

  - Aloe Vera Cream by California Baby
    Manufacturer Web site: *www.californiababy.com*
  - Calming Soothing & Healing Spray by California Baby
    Manufacturer Web site: *www.californiababy.com*

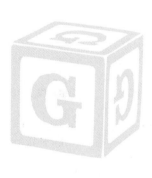
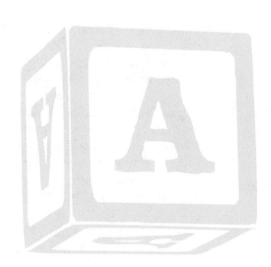

Chapter 20
Products for Nursing Mothers

Nursing should be a comfortable and enjoyable experience for both Mom and baby. Listed are key products to help you attain that goal. If you have the right breast pump and accessories, you can eliminate many of the problems that can occur during the breastfeeding experience.

BREAST PUMPS

A breast pump is a great thing to have for several reasons. It allows you to pump milk for your baby so someone else can take care of feedings if you're tired, sleeping, or away from your baby for more than three or four hours. Pumping after nursing completely empties your breasts, which signals your body to produce more milk. Pumping your breasts also allows you to use breast milk as a supplement if one is needed, which is a particular benefit for a mother of multiples.

Before you buy a pump, I suggest you rent the Medela Classic Breast Pump, which is a top-of-the-line pump, from your local hospital. Then, if all goes well—you produce enough milk and your baby is a good nurser—you might want to consider buying a breast pump.

There are three types of breast pumps:

1. Piston electric—efficient and easy to use, with various suction settings for your pumping comfort.
2. Mini electric—lightweight and convenient for traveling, but somewhat less efficient than the piston electric pump.
3. Manual—less expensive, but slow and not very practical.

You'll want to look for the following features when you buy a breast pump:

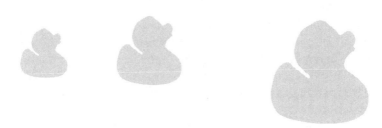

✔ Double-pumping capability. This feature cuts pumping time in half; pumping both breasts at the same time takes about twelve minutes.

✔ Adjustable suction levels. This feature provides more options for your comfort.

✔ Efficiency. Look for a pump that sucks more times per minute (known as the cycling time).

✔ Easy assembly. Fewer parts means easier assembly, a plus if you have to carry the pump around.

✔ Ease of use. Look for a pump that's easy to use, easy to clean, easy to carry, and compact and quiet.

○ Top-of-the-Line Electric Breast Pumps
Top-of-the-line breast pumps combine the features of hospital-grade pumps and the more portable breast pumps. They weigh approximately eight pounds. Top-of-the-line breast pumps are fully automatic, with quick cycling times, adjustable suction levels, and double-pumping capability. They usually come in attractive carrying cases that include storage bags, labels, clips, bottles, and nipple lotion. You can run most top-of-the-line electric pumps on a car lighter with an adapter that's sold separately. Some of these pumps even have built-in battery packs.

● Lactina Select Breast Pump by Medela
Manufacturer Web site: *www.medela.com*
Lactina breast pumps are ideal for long-term and frequent pumping, making them a favorite of working mothers. For the ultimate in pumping comfort and efficiency, the Lactina Select

allows you to select both the speed of the pump and the amount of vacuum power. For the mom-on-the-go, the PowerPak makes the Lactina usable when electric outlets are not available. This option includes a rechargeable battery and an adapter for use in a vehicle.

- Pump In Style Advanced Breast Pump by Medela

  Manufacturer Web site: *www.medela.com*

  This is the highest performing retail pump available, and the only electric retail pump with Natural Expression pumping for maximum milk flow. Natural Expression incorporates an advanced pumping pattern that mimics a baby's nursing rhythm by pumping in two distinct modes, let-down mode (simulates your baby's initial rapid sucking to initiate faster milk flow) and expression mode (simulates your baby's slower, deeper sucking for maximum milk flow in less time).

I've used the Pump In Style Advanced Breast Pump for both my babies and it works like a champ. I get plenty of milk quickly. It works just as well as the hospital-grade rented pumps. I highly recommended it to all breastfeeding mothers.—Hilary

- Whisper Wear Double Breast Pump

  Manufacturer Web site: *www.whisperwear.com*

  Whisper Wear is the world's first hands-free breast pump. Pump anytime, anywhere! Whisper Wear lets you get up and move around or even tend to your baby while you're pumping. Whisper Wear fits right into your bra under everyday clothing. It is soft, comfortable, gentle, and completely portable, operating with just two AA batteries. The soft breast cup and electronically controlled pump mimics the feel and sucking pattern of a baby. The small carry bag is lightweight and has a contemporary design. The pump also can be powered from any wall outlet or vehicle power outlet.

○ Mini Electric Breast Pumps

If you have to leave your baby for a few hours or even for a few days, the mini electric pumps are ideal.

- Double Select Breast Pump by Medela

  Manufacturer Web site: *www.medela.com*

The Double Select is a fully automatic double pump for short-term separation. This pump is lightweight, compact, and completely portable, with adjustable vacuum control, so traveling is convenient.

○ Manual Breast Pumps
Manual breast pumps are a lot slower and less efficient than electric breast pumps, but when necessary they can get the job done. Manual pumping is a quick, easy way to express milk when you have infrequent separations from your baby.

● ISIS On-the-Go Breast Pump by Avent
Manufacturer Web site: *www.aventamerica.com*
This pump set contains everything you need to maintain your milk supply and to express and store your breast milk when you are away from your baby.

● The SpringExpress Breastpump by Medela
Manufacturer Web site: *www.medela.com*
This convenient, portable manual pump is designed for moms who nurse their babies for most feedings. It is upgradable to electric or battery pumping with separate conversion kit.

BREAST-PUMP ACCESSORIES

Breast-pump accessories can get lost or broken, so it's nice to know where to go to find extra or replacement pieces.

○ Extra Breast Shield System
It's nice to have a few extra breast shield systems on hand. That way, you can avoid having to wash the same shield(s) after each pumping. Breast shield systems attach to the breast pump and allow milk to flow from the breast into a bottle.

● PersonalFit Breast Shield System by Medela
Manufacturer Web site: *www.medela.com*
This unique two-piece system lets moms choose the best breast-shield size for maximum personal comfort while they're pumping.

● PersonalFit Connectors by Medela
Manufacturer Web site: *www.medela.com*
The PersonalFit connectors will fit any Medela PersonalFit breast shield.

● Standard Breastshield by Medela
Vendor Web site: *www.breastfeed-essentials.com*
This shield is for use with all Medela breast pumps except the Little Hearts line.

○ Extra Valve/Membrane Assembly by Medela
These little pieces can easily get lost when you're washing the breast pump unit, so keep a few extra valve/membranes on hand.

- Extra Valves & Membranes by Medela
  Manufacturer Web site: *www.medela.com*
  The Valve/Membrane Assembly completes the standard breast shield and also accommodates the SoftFit and PersonalFit breast shields. These assemblies are necessary for the operation of all pumps.

○ Extra Tubing by Medela
  The tubing on the Medela breast pumps is not expensive to replace, and several different tubes are available to fit the various breast pumps.

  - Tubing for Medela Breast Pumps
    Vendor Web site: *www.mybreastpump.com*
    This Web site shows all the different tubing available from Medela and which Medela breast pumps the tubing fits.

○ Breast Milk Collection and Storage Bags
  Your breast milk is precious fluid, and storing it properly means protecting nutrients and antibodies. Store your breast milk in presterilized bags. Always mark the date and time of storage on the bag, and then fill it with the desired amount of milk, seal, and place in the freezer or refrigerator.

  - Breastmilk Storage Bags by Lansinoh
    Manufacturer Web site: *www.lansinoh.com*
    These bags are specially designed with a convenient pouring spout for transferring milk into a bottle. The double-zipper closure changes color when it's closed properly.

I really love these bags. The double-zipper closure reduces accidental spills. The bags are sterile and made from medical grade plastic, which is safer for milk storage. They freeze and thaw well too.—Annie

  - Collection Bags by Whisper Wear
    Manufacturer Web site: *www.whisperwear.com*
    Use these bags to collect and store up to 4 ounces of milk in the refrigerator or freezer. No-spill, sterilized collection bags have "oz." and "cc" markings.

  - CSF Breastmilk Storage Bags by Medela
    Manufacturer Web site: *www.medela.com*
    These bags are compatible with all Medela breast pumps for pumping directly into the bag. The special plastic retains breast milk's beneficial properties. The bags come with twist ties for easy storage and opening.

- Seal 'n Go Breast Milk Storage Bags by Gerber
  Manufacturer Web site: www.gerber.com
  These storage bags fit all disposable bottles. The self-standing bags make filling easier, and the zipper seal prevents the bags from leaking.

○ Storage Clips and Labels
  Airtight clips secure the storage bags you use for expressed breast milk. You can use one of the handy fill-in labels to add the time and date.

- Storage Clips and Labels by Avent
  Vendor Web site: *www.babybungalow.com*

○ Cleaning Products
  These products quickly and effectively clean breast-pump and feeding accessories at home or on the go.

- Cavacide—Germicidal Cleaner for Nonporous Surfaces by Medela
  Manufacturer Web site: *www.medela.com*
  Cavacide germicidal spray is ideal for daily, routine external cleaning of Medela electric breast pumps, vacuum pumps, baby scales, BiliBeds, and other surfaces that come in contact with skin.

- Quick Clean Breastpump and Accessory Wipes by Medela
  Manufacturer Web site: *www.medela.com*
  Unique wipes allow easy and convenient cleaning without soap and water. Wipes can be used anywhere—ideal for in the car, at work, travel, and more. Wipes are unscented and alcohol and bleach free. Just one wipe cleans both breastshields, valves, and membranes.

- Quick Clean Micro-Steam Bags by Medela
  Manufacturer Web site: *www.medela.com*
  These bags are a safe and easy way to clean breast pump parts. They eliminate 99.9 percent of all harmful bacteria and germs from most breast-pump parts and feeding accessories. To use, just add water and then heat in the microwave.

With Quick Clean Micro-Steam Bags, all you need is access to water and a microwave. Much faster than washing parts by hand. Directions are printed right on the bag.—Abby

○ Vehicle Lighter Adapter
  When you need to pump breast milk in the car, power your pump from your vehicle power outlet.

- Vehicle Lighter Adapter by Medela
  Manufacturer Web site: *www.medelausa.com*
- Whisper Wear Vehicle Adapter
  Manufacturer Web site: *www.whisperwear.com*

NURSING PADS

Many products are available that help make the nursing experience more comfortable and enjoyable. Nursing pads protect your clothing from messy leaks that can cause embarrassing stains. Nursing pads also help prevent sore nipples by drawing moisture away from the skin. There are two types of nursing pads: washable and disposable.

○ Washable Nursing Pads
- Lace Washable Bra Pads by Medela
  Manufacturer Web site: *www.medela.com*
  These pads have four layers: a lace outer layer, a waterproof layer, an absorbent layer, and an inner layer of soft, brushed flannel. The pads are seamless and contoured to avoid the bunched-up appearance of flat pads.
- Washable Breast Pads by Avent
  Manufacturer Web site: *www.aventamerica.com*
  The soft, brushed cotton lining of these pads is gentle against the skin. Their attractive lacy outer layer gives a more feminine appearance and prevents slippage.
- Washable Nursing Pads by Lansinoh
  Manufacturer Web site: *www.lansinoh.com*
  These pads' patented contour shape provides extra layers and the pads are preshrunk for an extra-smooth fit.

○ Disposable Nursing Pads
- Disposable Bra Pads by Medela
  Manufacturer Web site: *www.medela.com*
  This new bra pad gives hours of protection and ensures a natural, discreet appearance under clothes by employing contoured pleats to help accentuate the feminine form.
- Disposable Nursing Pads by Lansinoh
  Manufacturer Web site: *www.lansinoh.com*
  Their special contour and nonslip adhesive tape keeps these pads in place. The pads are individually wrapped for cleanliness and convenience.
- Disposable Lanolin Treated Nursing Pads by The First Years
  Manufacturer Web site: *www.thefirstyears.com*

These disposable breast pads have baby-safe lanolin built right in. The contoured, shaped nursing pads provide the soothing comfort and moisturizing power of lanolin without the mess of having to apply it.

- Premium Contoured Nursing Pads by Gerber
  Manufacturer Web site: *www.gerber.com*
  These pads' LeakSafe design draws liquid away from the skin and locks it in to prevent leaks. The pads are available in light, medium, or heavy flow design.
- Ultra Comfort Disposable Breast Pads by Avent
  Manufacturer Web site: *www.aventamerica.com*
  The ultra-soft top layer with its nipple indent keeps the breast dry at all times.

NIPPLE LOTIONS, CREAMS, AND THERAPY PACKS

Don't let sore or cracked nipples get in the way of breastfeeding your baby. You can use nipple lotions and creams to help prevent or soothe and heal sore or cracked nipples. These products are all hypoallergenic and preservative free. Use these products after every breastfeeding. There's no need to wash them off because they're safe for baby to ingest.

○ Nipple Lotions and Creams

If you're a nursing mother you shouldn't be without nipple lotion or cream. There are several good ones on the market that will protect your nipples from getting cracked and sore.—Molly

- Breast Therapy Gentle Moisturizing Balm by Gerber
  Manufacturer Web site: *www.gerber.com*
  Breast Therapy Gentle Moisturizing Balm is great for tender, chapped nipples.
- Lansinoh Lanolin for Breastfeeding Mothers
  Manufacturer Web site: *www.lansinoh.com*
  Lansinoh Lanolin is the only topical endorsed by La Leche League International in the United States.
- PureLan 100 by Medela
  Manufacturer Web site: *www.medela.com*
  PureLan 100 creates a moisture barrier to allow the skin to rehydrate from within.

○ Breast Therapy Warm/Cold Packs
Use heated therapy packs for engorgement, mastitis (an infection of the milk ducts in the breast), plugged ducts, and to encourage milk flow. Use cold therapy packs to relieve soreness and swelling.

- Breast Therapy Warm or Cool Relief Packs by Gerber
  Manufacturer Web site: *www.gerber.com*

○ Breast Shells

- Isis Comfort Breast Shell Set by Avent
  Manufacturer Web site: *www.aventamerica.com*
  The set includes two ventilated breast shells, two breast milk saver shells, and two ultra-soft silicone backing cushions. You wear the two different shells inside your bra and over your nipples. The ventilated breast shells have holes that provide exposure to air while they create a barrier between sore nipples and clothing to aid in the healing process. The breast-milk saver shells, without holes, collect leaking milk and also help prevent embarrassing wet spots. You can use the ultrasoft silicone backing cushions with both shells; the cushions have petal-like massagers that gently provide added stimulation to relieve engorgement. An extra-wide opening for the nipple provides comfort and actually helps to draw out inverted or flat nipples.

○ Nipple Shields
Nipple shields protect sore, cracked nipples while your baby is nursing. Nipple shields offer maximum comfort for mothers who have babies with latch-on difficulties. The shields are worn over the nipple and areola, which allows an uninterrupted flow of breast milk, while they provide a larger surface for baby to latch onto.

- Nipple Protectors by Avent
  Manufacturer Web site: *www.aventamerica.com*
  These shields are butterfly-shaped to allow your baby more contact with your breast. Baby can feel and smell your skin while nursing and will return more easily to the breast once your nipples are healed.

- Nipple Shields by Medela
  Manufacturer Web site: *www.medela.com*
  This nipple shield has an open section that lets your baby stay in touch with your familiar smell.

○ Inverted Nipple Products
Inverted nipples can make it difficult for your baby to latch onto your breast. These products will draw your nipples out so baby can secure a good latch.

- SoftShells Breast Shells by Medela
  Manufacturer Web site: *www.medela.com*
  SoftShells Breast Shells were created for the working mother. Offering the same care for sore, flat, or inverted nipples as Medela's other

shells, the SoftShells also offer increased comfort and a more flattering appearance.

- TheraShells Breast Shells by Medela
  Manufacturer Web site: *www.medela.com*
  TheraShells helps soothe sore nipples and flat or inverted nipples. They help keep nipples dry and prevent irritation, and the vented fronts provide air flow for healing and comfort.

NURSING STOOLS, PILLOWS, AND BIBS

○ Nursing Stools
You will spend the majority of your time feeding your baby. Whether you're breast- or bottle-feeding, a nursing stool makes the process more comfortable. A nursing stool elevates your legs so you can achieve just the right feeding angle and reduce the strain on your back, legs, shoulders, and arms. Using a nursing stool can also help ease the pain of an episiotomy or cesarean by taking pressure off those areas.

- NursingStool by Medela
  Manufacturer and Vendor Web sites: *www.medela.com*; *www.target .com*
  This little nursing stool comes in natural oak or white finish to complement any nursery.

- Nursing Stool by Kidcraft (various color options)
  Vendor Web site: *www.lullabylane.com*
  This stool has three comfortable positions for mom to rest her feet while nursing.

- Rock N Soft Cushioned Nursing Stool by Leachco
  Manufacturer Web site: *www.leachco.com*
  This stool's fleece-lined foot section keeps feet warm on cold nights.

○ Nursing Pillows
Nursing pillows make feeding your baby more manageable and comfortable. A nursing pillow lets you position your baby for the best possible latch-on and takes strain and pressure off your back, shoulders, arms, and neck.

- Boppy Nursing Pillow by Boppy
  Manufacturer Web site: *www.boppy.com*
  You can use the Boppy Nursing Pillow in many ways. You can use it as a nursing pillow or to prop infants up under an activity center, so they are not lying flat after they eat. You can use the pillow for tummy-time play and to help support baby while she's learning to sit up. The pillow is also great for simultaneously bottle-feeding multiples.

- My Brest Friend Feeding Pillow by Zenoff
  Vendor Web sites: *www.babiesrus.com*; *www.babyant.com*; *www.baby universe.com*

Moms love this versatile feeding pillow, which is perfect for nursing a single baby or twins. The pillow has adjustable Velcro straps to hold it in place. A built-in pocket holds bottles, diapers, TV remote, and other necessities.

- Natural Boost Adjustable Nursing Pillow by Leachco
  Manufacturer Web site: *www.leachco.com*
  Feeding baby at the right angle means less air in his tummy. Natural Boost adds that extra lift newborns need when you're breastfeeding.

○ Nursing Pillows for Twins

- "EZ-2-Nurse Twins" by Double Blessings
  Manufacturer Web site: *www.doubleblessings.com*
  The "EZ-2-Nurse Twins" nursing pillow is designed to allow Mother to nurse her babies from birth to two years of age. The pillow is angled in so babies safely roll toward their mother while they're nursing.

- Nurse EZ Twin Nursing Pillow by Basic Comfort
  Vendor Web site: *www.showeryourbaby.com*
  Nurse your babies together while your hands remain free. This nursing pillow comes with a separate back-support pillow that you can use wherever you need a little extra support for your lower back, upper back, or behind your head.

○ Nursing Bibs
When you're nursing, creating a private place isn't always easy. A nursing bib offers a discreet, comfortable way to nurse your baby.

- Covered 'N Cool Breastfeeding Cover by Leachco
  Manufacturer Web site: *www.leachco.com*
  The breastfeeding cover is made of 100 percent polyester mesh fabric so you will stay cool and comfortable while you're feeding your baby.

- Nursing Bib by Basic Comfort
  Manufacturer Web site: *www.basiccomfort.com*
  This bib is easy to put on and take off, with one snap. Special mesh around the neck allows for airflow and viewing.

OTHER NURSING ACCESSORIES

○ Nursing Breast Pad Case

- Nursing Breast Pad Case by Basic Comfort
  Vendor Web site: *www.babyabby.com*
  This handy carrying case has two compartments for clean and dirty breast pads. After you stop nursing, use the case as a change purse or cosmetic case.

○ Nursing Pillow Covers
Nursing pillow covers make it easy to keep your nursing pillow clean at all times. If the cover gets dirty, just remove it, wash it, and replace it.

- Boppy Slipcover by Boppy
  Manufacturer Web site: *www.boppy.com*
  The Boppy Slipcover is just like a pillowcase, fitting snugly over your existing Boppy.

- Extra Cover for "EZ-2-Nurse Twins" Foam Pillow by Double Blessings
  Manufacturer Web site: *www.doubleblessings.com*
  Slip this cover over the nursing pillow to keep the pillow clean and dry.

○ Hands-Free Pumping Attachments
Busy moms can answer the phone, read a book, work on the computer, or do other simple activities while they're using a breast pump with one of these attachments.

- Pumping Free Attachment Kit by Medela
  Vendor Web sites: *www.breastfeed-essentials.com*; *www.nurturecenter.com*
  With hands-free double pumping, the patented Pumping Free Attachment Kit is designed to provide exceptional convenience for busy mothers. When the attachment is fastened onto Medela's nursing bras, this unique product allows mothers to connect to a Medela electric breast pump (the Mini Electric and Double Pumping Mini Electric do not work with this attachment) and pump both breasts simultaneously, leaving both hands completely free. The Pumping Free Attachment Kit must be used with Medela Standard breast shields (it's not compatible with PersonalFit or SoftFit breast shields).

- Pumpin' Pal
  Manufacturer Web site: *www.pumpinpal.com*
  Pumpin' Pal fits all leading brands of breast pumps. This attachment is comfortable, easy to use, and adjusts to any body shape and size. Its use does not require the removal of shirt or bra.

Chapter 21
Feeding Time

Feeding time happens often during baby's first days and weeks. You'll want to be prepared from the start with all the right bottles, nipples, and other accessories that you'll need so you can focus your energies on baby during these special times of the day.

BOTTLES

Which bottle to use? There are many different types of bottles to choose from, and some are better than others. You can choose from the good old streamlined bottle, wide-mouth bottles, and a variety of disposable bottles. You also have a choice of plastic or glass. Glass bottles are heavy, and they're more likely to chip or break; plastic bottles are unbreakable and lightweight, and when baby is ready to feed himself, they are easy to hold.

When you're selecting bottles, keep in mind that they all come with different types of nipples, and the nipple that comes with the bottle might not be the right one for your baby. Babies can be very particular about the nipple they will accept. You sometimes have to experiment with several different types of nipples before you find the right one.

If you decide on the Avent, Playtex, or other wide-mouth bottles, you are limited to using only the types of nipples that fit these brands because of the wide ring. The ring is the piece that the nipple fits into and attaches to the bottle. If you select a streamlined bottle with a smaller ring, you will have a much broader range of nipples to choose from and for your baby to experiment with. For instance, if you buy the Classic Nurser by Evenflo and your baby doesn't like the nipple that comes with that bottle, you can buy other brands of nipples to try that will fit in the Evenflo ring.

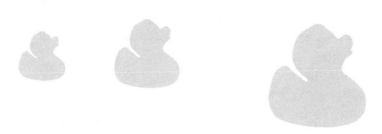

The number of bottles you'll need for a single baby is twelve; for twins, twenty-four; and for triplets, thirty.

NIPPLES

Nipples come in many shapes, sizes, and flow speeds (slow, medium, and fast). You can choose latex, silicone, or rubber nipples. Latex nipples are softer and more flexible, but they don't last long. Silicone nipples are firmer and hold their shape longer, but they tend to collapse when baby is feeding. Rubber nipples hold their shape, don't collapse, and last longer. Your baby will ultimately decide which nipple to use.

Begin by purchasing the smallest-sized nipple in a variety of types, and let your baby decide which one works best. You have your choice of traditional, orthodontic, or flat-topped nipples. Orthodontic nipples, designed to accommodate your child's palate and gums, have a bulb that's flat on one side. This flat side rests on your child's tongue. Flat-topped nipples emulate the shape of a mother's breast.

Caring for nipples is easy. Before you use store-bought nipples for the first time, boil them for five minutes. After that, you can wash the nipples in hot soapy water, rinse them well, and let them dry. As you're washing the nipples, be sure to squeeze water through the nipple hole to wash out any milk that might clog the hole. Don't soak nipples in soapy water for any length of time because they will get gummy, and you'll have to throw them out. Also, you may not want to wash nipples in the dishwasher because the soap does not always wash out thoroughly.

You can find Avent, Dr. Brown, Evenflo, Gerber, Munchkin, and Playtex bottles and nipples at your local drugstores, grocery stores, and baby specialty stores.

○ Clear Plastic, Streamlined, Reusable Bottles
   A streamlined bottle is straight from top to bottom, with no bends or indentations. A streamlined bottle has a smaller nipple ring than a wide-mouth bottle, which, as mentioned previously, lets you experiment with different types of nipples if you need to. Clear plastic bottles have easy-to-read ounce markings.

   ● Classic Clear Nursers by Evenflo
      Manufacturer Web site: *www.evenflo.com*

   ● Clear View Nurser by Gerber
      Manufacturer Web site: *www.gerber.com*

I love these Clear View Nursers. They are so easy to use, and if your baby doesn't like the nipple that comes on the bottle, you can easily try other nipples in the Gerber ring. —Molly

○ Nipples for Classic Streamlined, Reusable Bottles
   ● Classic Custom Flow Nipples by Evenflo
      Manufacturer Web site: *www.evenflo.com*
      The soft, flexible design of these nipples responds to baby's pressure to dispense just the right amount of liquid. Micro air vents allow air to return to the bottle, preventing nipple collapse and keeping air out of baby's tummy. Evenflo nipples ensure the right flow rate based on baby's age and nutritional needs.

   ● Classic Clear Silicone Nipples
      Slow, medium, and fast flow

   ● Classic Latex Nipples
      Slow, medium, and fast flow

   ● Classic Silicone Orthodontic Nipples
      Slow and medium flow

   ● Gerber Clear View Nurser Nipples
      Manufacturer Web site: *www.gerber.com*
      Gerber offers a wide variety of traditional nipples to fit your baby's needs.

   ● Latex Nipples
      Three-hole design comes with most standard Gerber bottles.

   ● Newborn Latex Nipples
      Specially designed for preemies and small babies.

- Nuk Orthodontic Body Vent Silicone or Latex Nipples, Size I
  Shaped like mother's nipple when she's breastfeeding, the body-vent nipple reduces swallowed air. Choose slow, medium, or fast flow.
- Silicone Nipples
  Choose slow, medium, or fast flow to fit baby's growing needs.

○ Wide-Mouth Reusable Bottles
  Wide-mouth bottles are easier to fill and clean, but, as mentioned previously, they have a large nipple ring that accommodates only the kind of nipple that fits that specific bottle. This design limits the kind of nipples you can use. If your baby doesn't like that particular kind of nipple and you have to experiment with other nipples, you'll need to buy another type of bottle.

- Avent Natural Feeding Bottle by Avent
  Manufacturer Web site: *www.aventamerica.com*
  Newborns fed with the Avent bottle reportedly had less colic and were more content when they were awake. The Avent bottle system has a patented antivacuum valve that prevents your baby from swallowing air, which causes painful gas. The Avent system may be a little difficult to start with for premature and small babies because of the amount of energy it takes to draw milk from the nipple. This effort tends to tire small babies, and they will eat less at each feeding.
- ComfortHold Bottles by Gerber
  Manufacturer Web site: *www.gerber.com*
  These bottles' unique triangular shape is designed to be easy for Mom and baby to hold. The soft-grip collar makes opening and closing the bottle easier.
- Elan Nursers by Evenflo
  Manufacturer Web site: *www.evenflo.com*
  This one-piece vent system prevents bubbles from entering the liquid and its one-piece design is easy to clean and maintain.
- Tri-Flow Wide Mouth Bottles by Munchkin
  Manufacturer Web site: *www.munchkininc.com*
  The Tri-Flow bottle lets you use one nipple for your baby's changing feeding needs; great for premature or small babies.

○ Nipples for Wide-Mouth Reusable Bottles
- Avent Anti-Colic Nipple
  Manufacturer Web site: *www.aventamerica.com*
  Avent teats are made from soft, pure, medical-grade silicone and shaped to mimic the breast in form and function. As your baby feeds, the patented anticolic skirt of the nipple flexes to allow air into the bottle and not your baby's stomach. The Clear Avent Anti-Colic Nipple should be used with the Natural Feeding Bottle and the VIA Nurser. Nipples are made in newborn-, slow-, medium-, and fast-flow versions.

- Comfort Latch Nipples by Gerber
  Manufacturer Web site: *www.gerber.com*
  These nipples are designed to provide a nursing experience that feels more like Mom. Comfort Latch Nipples's soft texture and natural shape make it easier for baby to latch on. Sure-flow vents ensure a smooth, consistent liquid flow for less air in baby's tummy.
- Elan Nipples by Evenflo
  Manufacturer Web site: *www.evenflo.com*
  The Elan silicone nipple has both textured and raised areas for improved latch-on. The nipple adjusts to baby's pressure for the right amount of liquid. The micro air vents balance air in the bottle and help prevent nipple collapse. These nipples are for use only with Elan products.
- Tri-Flow Wide Mouth Nipples by Munchkin
  Manufacturer Web site: *www.munchkininc.com*
  The Tri-Flow nipple system offers three flow rates—slow, medium, and fast flow—in one adjustable nipple to meet your baby's feeding needs. With a simple twist of the Tri-Flow nipple ring, you can control the flow of liquid so it's more like Mom's: slow for babies up to three months old, medium for three months to six months, or fast for babies six months and older. The wide, soft nipple promotes latch-on and suckling.

○ Dr. Brown's Bottles
   Dr. Brown bottles are wonderful, especially if you have a fussy, colicky baby who gets gas when she's feeding. Designed by a doctor, this revolutionary bottle helps reduce colic, burping, spitting up, and gas. A special internal vent prevents air bubbles from forming in liquids and keeps nipples from collapsing, which helps colicky babies settle down and sleep more comfortably. The vent also helps prevent fluid from gathering in baby's ears while she's feeding, which reduces the chance of painful ear infections. Each bottle comes with a silicone nipple, nipple collar, nipple cover, travel disc, and two-piece, snap-together vent.

Our twins had few issues with gas, have had no ear infections, and have done very well using these bottles. The Dr. Brown's system seems to really work!—Cara

- Dr. Brown's Natural Flow Bottle
  Vendor Web sites: *www.babybungalow.com*; *www.babycenter.com*; *www.kidsurplus.com*
- Dr. Brown's Natural Flow Wide Neck Bottle
  Vendor Web sites: *www.babybungalow.com*; *www.babycenter.com*; *www.kidsurplus.com*

○ Dr. Brown's Replacement Nipples

Dr. Brown's Replacement Nipples are for use with Dr. Brown's Natural Flow baby bottle and will allow your baby to enjoy the maximum benefits of the bottle. Only Dr. Brown's nipples should be used with the Dr. Brown's bottle. Nipples are made of silicone and will fit the 4-ounce and 8-ounce bottles. Nipples are available in three different sizes (levels 1, 2, and 3) to accommodate your growing baby. Use level 1 for newborns, level 2 for babies three months and up, and level 3 for more aggressive eaters.

- Dr. Brown's Nipples (Natural Flow and Wide Neck Nipples)
  Vendor Web sites: *www.babybungalow.com*; *www.babycenter.com*; *www .kidsurplus.com*

○ Soothie Bottle and Nipples

- Soothie Bottle by The First Years
  Vendor Web site: *www.soothie-pacifier.com*
  The Soothie Bottle has the same nipple shape and feel as the popular Soothie pacifiers distributed in hospitals nationwide. The convenient wide-neck design makes the bottle easy to clean.

- Soothie Stage 1 Nipple by The First Years
  Vendor Web site: *www.soothie-pacifier.com*
  Soothie replacement nipples are made of medical-grade silicone. They come in slow/medium flow and medium/fast flow.

DISPOSABLE BOTTLES

With these bottles, you simply insert a presterilized liner into the bottle and fill the liner with breast milk or formula. As your baby feeds, the liner contracts to minimize air intake that can cause painful gas and other stomach discomforts. When baby is finished, throw the liner away. A disadvantage of these bottles is that you have to continuously buy new liners. And because the liner contracts as baby feeds, it's hard to tell how much she has actually consumed during a feeding. Disposable bottles come with a wide-mouth ring, so you have to use the nipple designated for that bottle. And if your baby doesn't like that nipple, you'll have to buy another type of bottle.

○ Disposable Bottle Holders, Bags, Liners, and Nipples

- Avent Disposable Bottle Holders, Bags, and Nipples
  Manufacturer Web site: *www.aventamerica.com*

- Avent Conventional Nurser
  Unique platform base supports bottle liner when you're filling it with breast milk or formula.

- The Breast Milk Storage Set
  Presterilized disposable bottle bags come with sealing clips and labels. Bags are great for storing expressed breast milk in the freezer.

- Blue Tinted Avent Nipples
  Use the Blue Tinted Avent Nipples with the Avent Conventional Nurser.
- Playtex Disposable Bottle System Holders
  Manufacturer Web site: *www.playtexbaby.com*
- Original Nurser
  The Original Nurser comes with a Latex Natural Action Infant Nipple.
- Premium Eazy-Feed Nurser
  With its built-in burping mechanism, the Eazy-Feed Nurser lets you easily rid the bottle of excess air before you feed baby.
- Premium Nurser
  With its natural-shape silicone nipple, the Premium Nurser eases baby's transition between breast and bottle. The contoured shape is easy for Mom to hold.
- Playtex Disposable Bottle Liners
  Manufacturer Web site: *www.playtexbaby.com*
  They are presterilized for convenience and cleanliness. Insert the liner in the bottle, fill, and you're ready to feed your baby.
- Drop-Ins Disposable Liners
  These bottle liners are preformed, so all you have to do is place one in a nurser and fill it. Twist on the nipple and ring, and you're done.
- Original Soft Bottle Liners
  The curved bottom of these liners allows for easy insertion into the holder. These liners are ideal for breast milk storage.
- Playtex Nipples
  Manufacturer Web site: *www.playtexbaby.com*
- NaturalLatch Nipple
  The stem of the NaturalLatch nipple elongates when baby sucks, similar to a mother's nipple during breastfeeding.
- NaturalLatch Silicone and NaturalLatch Latex Nipples
  The Playtex NaturalLatch nipple is a perfect choice for babies who are switching between bottle and breast. To reduce nipple confusion, the NaturalLatch nipple features a textured area that is more like the breast. The NaturalLatch nipples have been clinically proven to support breastfeeding. The nipples are available in slow, fast, and tri-cut flow rates.
- Orthodontic Nipple
  This medium-flow latex nipple's shape promotes healthy oral development for babies.

HANDS-FREE BABY BOTTLES WITH NIPPLE SYSTEMS

With a hands-free bottle, you can feed baby in an upright position just about anywhere—in a car seat, bouncy seat, swing, stroller, front carrier, backpack, exersaucer, or grocery seat. A hands-free bottle is a must for moms of multiples: no more feeding one baby while the others cry. Now everyone can eat at the same time.

○ Hands-Free Bottle Systems

- Hands-Free Baby Feeding System by Podee
  Manufacturer Web site: *www.podee.com*
  The Podee Baby Feeding System includes an 8-ounce bottle and all the other required components. This feeding system enables baby to feed in an upright and semiupright position, as recommended by pediatricians, to help prevent ear infections. Eating in this position also helps prevent colic. The system converts to a toddler bottle so the toddler can drink the fluid without looking upward. Extra replacement tubes and nipples are available.

- Pacifeeder by Pacifeeder
  Manufacturer Web site: *www.pacifeeder.com*
  The Pacifeeder promotes doctor-recommended semiupright feeding positions to help prevent ear infections. The strap helps Pacifeeder attach to any car seat, stroller, or baby carrier. The Smart Flow system adjusts flow based on baby's needs and prevents the nipple from leaking. Pacifeeder's nipple stays full of liquid until the bottle is empty, to reduce ingestion of air and thus reduce the chance of colic. Using any standard nipple, you can quickly convert Pacifeeder to a regular baby bottle.

BOTTLE AND NIPPLE ACCESSORIES

○ Bottle and Nipple Brush
  Scrub bottles and nipples clean with a bottle and nipple brush. The bottle brush gets all the milk residue out, while the nipple brush ensures that any clogs are removed so that fresh milk will flow freely during a feeding.

- Bottle and Nipple Brush by Gerber
  Vendor Web site: *www.kidsurplus.com*
  The large brush cleans bottles effectively while the small one reaches into nipples.

- Deluxe Bottle Brush by Munchkin
  Manufacturer Web site: *www.munchkininc.com*
  The suction-cup base keeps the brush standing upright to air dry and avoid contact with germs.

- Floating Bottle Brush by Mommy's Helper
  Vendor Web sites: *www.babybungalow.com*; *www.kidsurplus.com*
  Floating Bottle Brushes have brush handles that are always visible—no more hunting under suds to find the brush. The brush has a sponge tip for cleaning hard-to-reach areas.

- Soap Dispenser Bottle and Nipple Brush by Sassy
  Manufacturer Web site: *www.sassybaby.com*
  This brush features a soap-dispensing reservoir with bottle and nipple scrubbers on opposite ends. The foam and bristle-head attachments are uniquely shaped for thorough bottle cleaning.

○ Dishwasher Basket for Nipples, Rings, and Caps
  Dishwasher baskets make cleaning nipples, rings, caps, pacifiers, feeding utensils, and teething toys more convenient. Some dishwasher baskets have one large compartment that holds everything, and others have a top compartment for nipples and a large bottom compartment for other feeding accessories.

  - Deluxe Dishwasher Basket by Munchkin
    Manufacturer Web site: *www.munchkininc.com*
    Two baskets in one: The top basket holds nipples, and the bottom basket holds pacifiers and accessories.

  - Infant Dishwasher Basket by Prince Lionheart
    Manufacturer Web site: *www.princelionheart.com*
    This is the only dishwasher basket that holds nipples directly above water jets for the most thorough sanitizing and rinsing.

  - Toddler Dishwasher Basket by Prince Lionheart
    Manufacturer Web site: *www.princelionheart.com*
    This is the largest dishwasher basket available. Everything goes in one compartment.

○ Drying Rack for Bottles, Nipples, Rings, Caps, and Pacifiers
  Don't worry about running your dishwasher just for bottles. Wash bottles, nipples, rings, caps, and pacifiers in hot, soapy water, rinse them well, and place them on the drying rack to drain and dry. Buy a drying rack that drains right into the sink so water doesn't puddle in the bottom of the drying rack or on your kitchen countertop.

  - Drain 'n Dry Bottle Drying Rack by Mommy's Helper
    Vendor Web sites: *www.babybungalow.com*; *www.babycatalog.com*
    This drying rack is easy to assemble; just snap the pegs into the holes. The waterfall lip hangs over the edge of the sink for easy water drainage.

  - The Complete Drying Station by Prince Lionheart
    Manufacturer Web site: *www.princelionheart.com*
    This is the only drying organizer that accommodates all sizes of cups, bottles, nipples, and cup parts. This product adjusts to fit all sinks and counters, and its slanted design allows for thorough draining and drying.

  - 2 in 1 Drying Rack by The First Years
    Vendor Web sites: *www.babiesrus.com*; *www.babyant.com*; *www.lullaby lane.com*

This rack is designed so all bottles are together and all rings and caps are together, which makes it easy to put them away or get at them quickly. The rack drains right into the sink.

○ Sterilizer

Pediatricians don't recommend sterilizing bottles and nipples anymore. The only time you really need a sterilizer is if you're going to travel and are not sure about the water conditions in that area. But if you feel you must sterilize your baby's bottles, here are two options:

- Express Electric Steam Sterilizer by Avent
  Manufacturer Web site: *www.aventamerica.com*
  This sterilizer is the safest and easiest way to sterilize breastfeeding and bottle-feeding equipment. Just add water and switch it on. The intensive heat of the steam kills all household bacteria in just nine minutes.

- Express Microwave Steam Sterilizer by Avent
  Manufacturer Web site: *www.aventamerica.com*
  The Express Microwave Steam Sterilizer uses the speed and convenience of your microwave to sterilize breastfeeding and bottle-feeding equipment safely and simply. The unit sterilizes up to four bottles and accessories in less than seven minutes. Its compact design and clip-on lid make it ideal for travel.

○ Bottle Warmer

A bottle warmer lets you warm baby's bottle and food jars any time during the day or night. The suggested bottle warmers warm all bottle styles—streamlined, wide mouth, and disposables. The warmers all have an automatic shut-off feature, so bottles and food jars never overheat.

Bottle warmers really help with middle of the night feedings. I don't have to run to the kitchen or bathroom for a cup of hot water.—Sherry

- Electronic Bottle and Food Warmer by Dex
  Manufacturer Web site: *www.dexproducts.com*
  This warmer is electronically controlled to never overheat. A pleasant chime sounds and a green light appears when the bottle is ready.

- Night & Day Bottle Warmer System by The First Years
  Manufacturer Web site: *www.thefirstyears.com*
  The Night & Day Bottle Warmer System is great, especially at night. There's no need to go to the kitchen. The thermal cooler keeps two prechilled bottles cold until they're needed. When it's time to feed,

simply take the bottle, put it in the warming chamber along with pre-measured water, and the bottle warms in minutes. A soft-glow night light provides enough light for nighttime feedings.

- Quick Serve Bottle Warmer by The First Years
  Manufacturer Web site: *www.thefirstyears.com*
  This compact bottle warmer is great for the nursery.

○ Baby Bottle and Food Carousels
Baby food carousels keep your kitchen counters neat and conserve cabinet space. The rotating shelves let you know what foods you have on hand and provide easy access to baby's meals.

- Baby's Feeding Center by Gerber
  Vendor Web sites: *www.babiesrus.com*; *www.kidsurplus.com*
  This carousel-style baby-food center can hold up to thirty-six jars of baby food, eight bottles, and formula.

- Baby Food Organizer by Munchkin
  Manufacturer Web site: *www.munchkininc.com*
  This organizer holds up to twenty-four baby food jars and has handy storage space for utensils.

- Pantry Organizer by Sassy
  Manufacturer Web site: *www.sassybaby.com*
  This carousel holds twenty-four jars or sixteen junior jars in the space of a nine-inch dinner plate.

- Universal Food Organizer by Prince Lionheart
  Manufacturer Web site: *www.princelionheart.com*
  This product is the only height-adjustable, stackable, revolving carousel. The distance between trays is adjustable to fit all sizes of containers.

USING POWDERED FORMULA

○ Powdered Formula
Powdered formula is most like breast milk. I recommend Enfamil with Iron or Nestlé Good Start. If your family has a history of milk allergies, be sure to ask your pediatrician which formula you should use.

○ 64-Ounce Calibrated Measuring Cup or Pitcher
If you are making a large amount of formula, you need a large measuring cup.

This size measuring cup is the best for mixing formula. I was able to make a whole day's worth of bottles for my twins in one batch and line them up in the fridge so we were always ready for the next feeding.—Dena

○ One-Cup (8 oz.) Calibrated Measuring Cup
If you are making a large amount of formula, use one cup plus one and one-half scoops of formula to 32 ounces of water.

○ Wire Whisk
Mixing powdered formula with a wire whisk will help break up clumps and prevent nipples from clogging.

Mixing Powdered Formula

Into a glass measuring cup, pour an amount of water equal to the amount of formula you wish to make. Heat the water in the microwave for two minutes or until it's hot (the powder will dissolve better in hot water). Open a can of powdered formula and remove the scoop. Put the lid back on and shake the can to loosen the powder; doing this makes it easier to fill the scoop. Tap the sides of the can before you remove the lid. Add one scoop of formula for every 2 ounces of water in the measuring cup, unless specified otherwise on the can or by your pediatrician. For instance, if you have 12 ounces of water, you would add six scoops of formula. After you measure out the formula, mix it into the water with a wire whisk. The whisk will break up the powder so you will have lump-free formula. Pour the mixed formula into bottles and refrigerate them. When baby is ready to eat, take a bottle from the refrigerator, warm it, and you're ready to feed baby.

It's best to mix enough formula for twenty-four hours. If you mix only enough for one bottle at a time, you'll have to shake the bottle to mix the formula, which causes a lot of air bubbles in the mixture. Then, when baby eats, the air bubbles will get into her tummy and cause gas.

FEEDING ACCESSORIES

Mealtime calls for several different feeding utensils. For example, you might want heat-sensitive spoons and bowls with a suction-cup base. Baby food processors make it easy to make your own baby food. You can even buy a bib that will hold the baby's bottle for you.

○ Temperature-Sensitive Feeding Spoons
When they're first learning to eat from a spoon, babies tend to bite down hard. Soft-bite spoons have a firm but soft coating, so they are gentle on baby's gums. The small bowl of the spoon is sized just right for first-time eaters, and its easy-grip handle make feeding time easier for Mom and Dad. The spoon's temperature-sensitive safety tip changes colors when the food is too hot.

When my baby started eating solid food I wanted to make sure I didn't give her anything that was too hot. These spoons turn white if food is too hot.—Leslie

- Easy-Grasp Soft-Bite Spoons by The First Years
  Manufacturer Web site: *www.thefirstyears.com*
- Safety Spoons by Munchkin
  Manufacturer Web site: *www.munchkininc.com*

○ Feeding Spoons Without a Temperature-Sensitive Safety Tip

- Soft Bite Infant Spoon by Gerber
  Manufacturer Web site: *www.gerber.com*
- Soft Bite Spoons by Evenflo
  Manufacturer Web site: *www.evenflo.com*
- Soft Bite Spoon by The First Years
  Manufacturer Web site: *www.thefirstyears.com*

○ Feeding Bowls with Suction-Cup Bases
Babies tend to throw everything on the floor, including their dishes. A suction-cup base will keep feeding bowls securely on the highchair tray or table.

- Feeding Bowl with Lid by Playtex
  Manufacturer Web site: *www.playtexbaby.com*
  These handy bowls with lids are great for serving, storing, and transporting your baby's meals when you're on the go.
- Smart Serve Suction Bowl by The First Years
  Manufacturer Web site: *www.thefirstyears.com*
  The food might not stay in the bowl, but at least these bowls will stay on the table. Textured handles make the bowls easy to hold, and the sure-fit lids won't leak; they stay on even if the bowl is dropped.
- Stay Put Divided Warming Dish by Munchkin
  Manufacturer Web site: *www.munchkininc.com*
  Fill the reservoir of this dish with hot water to keep baby's food nice and warm. Three divided sections give you plenty of space for all of baby's foods. The suction-cup base holds the dish firmly in place.
- Warming Dish by Sassy
  Manufacturer Web site: *www.sassybaby.com*
  This warming dish keeps baby's food warm without cords or plugs. Just add warm water through the spout to keep food warm during mealtime.

○ Baby-Food Processor
Now preparing fresh, healthy baby food is simple and easy. There's no more need to buy expensive commercial baby food when you can make your own in seconds. This way, baby eats the same nutritious foods as the rest of the family.

- Baby Food Chopper by Munchkin
  Vendor Web site: *www.munchkininc.com*

This electric chopper transforms fresh food into nutritious baby food. The one-touch action purées, grinds, or chops. The chopper contains an easy-pour spout and stainless steel blade and comes with a recipe book.

- Baby Food Preparer by Bebesounds
  Vendor Web site: *www.greatbabyrooms.com*
  This all-in-one food preparer grinds, strains, grates, juices, and purées so you can easily make fresh food for your baby at home or on the go.

- Electric Baby Food Processor by Dex
  Manufacturer Web site: *www.dexproducts.com*
  This processor makes healthy and fresh baby food instantly, and its convenient mixing/serving bowl makes cleanup a snap.

- BabySteps Electric Food Mill by KidCo
  Manufacturer Web site: *www.kidco.com*
  Blends and purées fresh foods into healthy meals for your baby.

○ Hands-Free Baby-Bottle Holder
This product is especially great for feeding multiples.

- The Bottle Bundle by Little Wonders
  Manufacturer Web site: *www.littlewonders.com*
  Invented by a mom, the Bottle Bundle is a soft, cuddly, U-shaped pillow with a fabric-covered elastic bottle holder. The unit securely holds your baby's bottle at the correct angle. You can use the Bottle Bundle while you're holding the baby or when he is in the bouncy seat, car seat, or stroller.

Chapter 22
Baby Gear

Whether you're looking to stimulate or soothe your baby, a wide variety of activity equipment is available to suit your needs. Exersaucers provide hours of stimulation and fun. Jumpers let baby exercise by bouncing and turning all around. Swings and bouncy seats soothe and calm baby when he's fussy.

Exersaucers

Exersaucers are a great source of entertainment for your baby. Babies love being upright so they can look around in all directions. Exersaucers can entertain any child who is old enough to sit up and control head movement, which usually means a baby four months old and older. You can fix the exersaucer seat in the stationary position or unlock it to swivel. Because the seat can swivel a full 360 degrees, your baby can keep you in sight at all times. Exersaucers are stationary. They have no wheels so baby can't roll around. Exersaucers let your baby bounce, spin, and rock without fear of tipping or tumbling down stairs. They are a confined, safe place to put your baby while you do housework or talk on the phone—as long as baby is in sight.

Exersaucers are made of durable molded plastic with a wide base and an adjustable seat in the center. Different models feature a variety of toys, music, and other gadgets to keep your baby entertained and stimulate hand-eye coordination, focus, and perception. A wide surrounding tray has plenty of room for toys and snacks. The height-adjustable seats accommodate your growing baby. Mechanisms stabilize the saucer base for younger babies. Take out the stops when your baby gets older so he can really rock. Seat cushions are easy to clean—just remove the seat cover and machine wash it. Exersaucers are perfect for indoor or outdoor use. When your

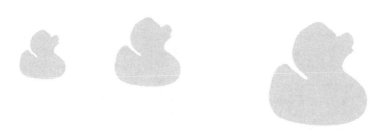

child is in an exersaucer, make sure that furniture, dangling appliance cords, curtain pulls, or hot surfaces such as ovens or radiators are out of reach.

○ Stationary Exersaucers

A stationary exersaucer is a fun alternative to a walker. It allows your baby the same active play and exercise as a walker with wheels, but it is safer because it's stationary. Baby can't maneuver to an unsafe area such as an incline or the top of the stairs. Even though the exersaucer is stationary, never leave your child unattended while she's in one.

My son loves his exersaucer. He can sit upright and see what's going on all around him. He loves to explore all the toys, listen to the music, and watch the lights. I can take him from room to room, get things done around the house, and know that he's safe and secure.—Barbara

- Discover & Play Activity Center by Baby Einstein
  Manufacturer Web site: *www.babyeinstein.com*
  This rocking activity center features nine engaging, interactive toys and classical melodies. It introduces animal sounds and names in Spanish and English, and exposes babies to colors, shapes, and textures.

- ExerSaucer SmartSteps Active Learning Center by Evenflo

  Manufacturer Web site: *www.evenflo.com*

  This activity center offers all the great features of Evenflo's line of exer-saucers, with the addition of removable, interactive learning toys. The electronic SmartSteps learning pod grows with your child by offering teethers and big buttons for younger babies, and simple word-association features for older babies. The removable electronic learning pod book has a volume control. The overhead electronic toy bar entertains baby with music and lights. The SmartSteps learning pod is also removable, and so it goes where baby goes. Use this learning pod in the activity center or on the floor for tummy-time fun.

- ExerSaucer Ultra 2-in-1 Active Learning Center by Evenflo

  Manufacturer Web site: *www.evenflo.com*

  The ExerSaucer Ultra has eleven age-appropriate toys and twenty-two songs to help baby achieve ten developmental milestones such as cause/effect understanding, musical development, and more. The unit folds flat for travel and storage, and its built-in carry handle makes it easy to transport.

- Intellitainer by Fisher Price

  Manufacturer Web site: *www.fisher-price.com*

  Learning can be fun for baby while he's sitting in a seat that slides back and forth and spins around. The Intellitainer features piano keys that light up and teach colors. It also includes a storybook that can tell nursery rhymes, a roller that sings the ABCs, and a school bus that sings about numbers.

Jumpers

Babies love to bounce and jump around. Doorway jumpers and floor jumpers are baby seats with springs that attach to a door frame or sit stationary on the floor. When your baby is strong enough to support himself on his feet, he's ready for a jumper. This ability usually occurs between five and six months of age. Playing in a jumper lets babies develop leg muscles and release pent-up energy. Standing up straight, they can use their legs to control their movement. Playing in the jumper develops coordination and keeps babies entertained until they are walking on their own.

○ Doorway Jumpers

Doorway jumpers are easy to install on most door frames. The straps should be wide and adjustable to make getting baby in and out easy. The seat should be removable for easy cleaning. Some jumpers have bumpers to reduce wear and tear on your doorway. A play tray can provide a place for toys and snacks.

- Bumper Jumper by Graco
  Manufacturer Web site: *www.gracobaby.com*
  The Bumper Jumper is great for getting your baby up and active. It comes with two soft, removable, interactive toys attached to adjustable play rings, so you can bring toys to baby's level. The bumpers protect your door frames from marring.
- ExerSaucer SmartSteps Jump & Go by Evenflo
  Manufacturer Web site: *www.evenflo.com*
  The SmartSteps Jump & Go has an electronic play station with lights, eight songs, and six activities. You can remove the play station for tummy-time play.

The Jump & Go is the only thing my active baby will sit in for more than ten minutes. She jumps in it and laughs the whole time. She loves it.—Sandy

○ Floor Jumper
  If you don't want to hang a jumper in a doorway, you can use a stationary floor jumper. A stationary floor jumper lets baby jump around and exercise anywhere in the house.
- Deluxe Jumperoo by Fisher Price
  Manufacturer Web site: *www.fisher-price.com*
  The Deluxe Jumperoo lets baby jump to her heart's delight, and the sturdy, freestanding steel frame helps keep baby safe while she's jumping. A removable, interactive toy tray rewards baby's jumping with lights and fun sounds. Remove the toy tray to reveal a snack tray underneath. The height of this jumper adjusts easily to custom fit your child.

Swings

A swing is a wonderful way to calm and soothe your baby. There are two types of swings: wind-up and battery powered. Wind-up swings run for fifteen to thirty minutes with a single winding, while battery-powered swings can run for hours and hours. I have listed only battery-operated swings here because they are much more practical to use.

FEATURES TO LOOK FOR

✔ Reclining seat—lets newborns sit in a semiupright position.
✔ Tip resistant—the wide base keeps the swing stable and safe.
✔ Washable seat cushions—for easy cleaning.
✔ Restraint strap—keeps baby securely in place.

✔ Lullaby tunes—introduce your child to the classics.

✔ Mobiles—focus your baby's attention.

✔ Soft toys—entertain and amuse.

✔ Open top design for easy access.

✔ Variable speed settings.

○ Battery-Operated Swings
Look for a swing with an open-top design, just like the recommended ones below. The open top makes getting baby in and out easy.

- Baby Einstein Discover & Play Swing by Graco
Manufacturer Web site: *www.gracobaby.com*
Baby Einstein Discover & Play Swing has a spiral mobile with three soft toys: a colorful ladybug, bee, and sun that bounce and spin with swing movement to provide overhead visual stimulation while baby is in the reclined position. The swing includes fifteen Baby Einstein lullaby melodies and five nature sounds to soothe and entertain baby. A removable, electronic Baby Einstein play tray introduces baby to animal names and sounds, dancing lights, and playtime melodies. The one-hand, four-position recline adjusts for your baby's comfort.

- Deluxe Flutterbye Dreams Swing by Fisher Price
Manufacturer Web site: *www.fisher-price.com*
The birdies' fluttering motion is so lifelike baby will be captivated by it. Baby's gentle swinging motion makes the birdie flutter overhead accompanied by music, sounds, and soft lights. Your baby can activate the lights, sounds, and music by pulling on one of the dangling toys, or you can activate the features for ten minutes of continuous play. When baby is ready to take a nap, you can swing the bar out of the way.

- Deluxe Quick Response Swing by Fisher Price
Manufacturer Web site: *www.fisher-price.com*
A remote control activates swinging, music, or both! Choose one of five different swinging speeds, or classical music and lullabies. The interactive, removable toy tray for sensory development fits over the snack tray. The swing also includes a multipurpose basket that holds all of baby's essentials.

- Lovin' Hug Swing by Graco
Manufacturer Web site: *www.gracobaby.com*
The Lovin' Hug Swing holds babies up to 30 pounds. The two-speed soothing vibration is located on the swing seat and operates with or without the swinging motion. Six speeds and fifteen classical and nature tunes allow you to choose the soothing experience that's just right for your baby. A four-position recline provides comfort and support.

- Nature's Touch Baby Papasan Cradle Swing by Fisher Price
  Manufacturer Web site: *www.fisher-price.com*
  With the touch of a button, you can swing baby in a cradle-like motion from side to side or a traditional back-and-forth motion. There are six soothing swing speeds and a cozy papasan seat that reclines to two different positions. A motorized mobile that spins overhead and a removable toy bar keep baby entertained as she swings.
- Ocean Wonders Aquarium Cradle Swing by Fisher Price
  Manufacturer Web site: *www.fisher-price.com*
  This swing features a cradle motion, which swings baby side to side, and a swing motion, which swings baby front to back. The push-button control turns the seat 90 degrees to switch from swing to cradle. An aquarium water globe has changing lights and swimming characters, and a mobile with four plush, aquatic friends keeps baby company.

My baby is super fussy. The Ocean Wonders Aquarium Cradle Swing is the only thing I can get her to sleep in. It is the best! I can actually get things done around the house.—Marie

- Swyngomatic Infant Swing by Graco
  Manufacturer Web site: *www.gracobaby.com*
  This is a great swing with lots of features. A detachable toy bar and a soft-covered mobile stimulate and entertain your baby, while fifteen classical lullaby tunes soothe him. Some models feature a forty-minute timer with four settings for automatic shut-off. The rotating toy bar makes getting baby in and out of the swing easy. Six speed settings let you select the right one for your baby's needs. The four-position reclining seat provides comfort and support for babies of all ages.
- Travel Swings
  Travel swings have all the features of a full-size swing in a portable, compact size. They are the perfect piece of play equipment to take wherever you go.
  - Aquarium Take-Along Swing by Fisher Price
    Manufacturer Web site: *www.fisher-price.com*
    This is a gentle, quiet swing with a seat level just right for newborns. The swinging motion makes fish in the colorful tank look like they're swimming. Eight different swing speeds will soothe your baby while

she's watching her fishy friends swim. And she can pull on the hanging sea-creature friends for music and dancing lights.

- Open Top Take-Along Swing by Fisher Price
  Manufacturer Web site: *www.fisher-price.com*
  This swing has five swing speeds and plays five different songs. Link-a-doos toys link easily to the swing-away toy bar or to the sides of the swing, where baby can reach them. The swing folds easily for travel.

- Take-Along Sensory Swing by Fisher Price
  Manufacturer Web site: *www.fisher-price.com*
  Miracles and Milestones toys on this swing stimulate baby's developing abilities throughout the early months. The toy bar features a cute black and white panda and mirror. Seven fun songs, sounds, and rattles, and noise-making toys encourage baby's auditory senses. There are five swing speeds as well. When you want to go out, you can fold up all that fun and go anywhere. Carry handles on each side let you carry the swing from room to room, even with baby in it.

○ Rocking Infant Seat
  Babies love to be soothed while being held in a gliding rocking chair. Now they can enjoy that same soothing motion in a reclining glider that's made just for them!

- Soothing Motions Glider by Fisher Price
  Manufacturer Web site: *www.fisher-price.com*
  The Soothing Motions Glider provides a gliding motion for baby in two ways—side to side or front to back. This glider is so plush and comfy you'll love putting your newborn in it right from the start. The glider has a recline position for newborns, and a slightly inclined position for older babies. As baby glides back and forth, you can choose from soothing or playful music, and she can gaze at the plush toys overhead.

Bouncy Seats

Bouncy seats buy parents blocks of time throughout the day. The vibrating motion calms and relaxes babies and often lulls them to sleep. You also can use them for baby to play in, and for feeding baby before she's ready for a highchair. If your baby has a reflux problem, doctors often recommend placing baby upright in a bouncy seat after she eats.

Babies love sitting in bouncy seats, especially if the seat vibrates. Place your baby in the bouncy seat in front of a sliding glass door or window on a windy day; the blowing trees and leaves will entertain her for hours. Or place the bouncy seat in front of the TV, where children can watch *Baby Einstein, Sesame Street,* and other children's shows.

You can put your newborn in a bouncy seat and still use the seat nine or ten months later. Most bouncers support a baby up to 25 pounds. Bouncy seats are lightweight, so you can carry them from room to room. An attachable toy bar provides entertainment and helps develop hand-eye coordination.

FEATURES TO LOOK FOR

✔ Machine-washable padding—makes cleaning much easier.

✔ Multiple vibration speeds—calms and soothes baby.

✔ Attachable toy bar—provides entertainment and helps develop hand-eye coordination.

✔ Extended leg room—more comfortable for little legs.

✔ Crotch strap—waist high to keep baby securely in the seat.

✔ Adjustable canopy—protects baby from the sun.

✔ Music and lights—provide visual and audio stimulation.

○ Bouncy Seats with Vibrations
  Look for a bouncy seat that has a gentle slope to the seat, like the ones following, so your newborn is not sitting in an uncomfortable upright position.

  ● Kick & Play Bouncer by Fisher Price
    Manufacturer Web site: *www.fisher-price.com*
    The toys found on the toy bar on this bouncer stimulate sight, sound, and touch. As baby kicks, lights twinkle, and one of fourteen different songs begins to play, along with eight whimsical sound effects. Baby's own movement activates a gentle bouncing motion, and you can switch on calming vibrations to soothe baby like a ride in the car does.

  ● Ocean Wonders Aquarium Bouncer by Fisher Price
    Manufacturer Web site: *www.fisher-price.com*
    This bouncer soothes baby with aquatic sights and sounds. Its bubble action makes starfish kiss and swim, and lights pulse overhead. The bouncer has two play modes: continuous and baby activated. There are also three songs and two aquatic sounds, a removable toy bar with toys to develop baby's senses, and calming vibrations.

  ● Sensory Selections Bouncer by Fisher Price
    Manufacturer Web site: *www.fisher-price.com*
    The Sensory Selection bouncer lets you choose which of baby's senses you want to stimulate. You can customize the bouncer to stimulate baby's sight with the overhead motorized mobile, baby's hearing with music and sound effects, or baby's touch with the textured toys that are right within his reach. Or you can choose any combination or all three! You can flip these components out of the way when it's time to relax.

○ Bouncenette

You can use a bouncenette as a bassinet, a bouncy seat, or a portable play area to provide hours of fun and a comfortable place for baby to take a nap. Music, lights, and motion calm baby if he's fussy. Toy bars provide entertainment and stimulate baby's senses. Lightweight and portable, a bouncenette is easy to take anywhere you go—it's the perfect piece of equipment to take when you're visiting Grandma or friends, or going to the park or the beach.

- Soothing Comfort Bouncenette by Safety 1st
  Manufacturer Web site: *www.safety1st.com*
  This bouncenette is perfect for naps, play, and taking baby outdoors. The Soothing Comfort Bouncenette combines all the great features of a bouncer and a portable bassinet. The quilted, reclining seat; gentle vibration; and nature sounds soothe baby at home and on the go.

HIGHCHAIRS

When your baby is sitting up and eating solid foods (around six or seven months of age), you will want to purchase a highchair. If your highchair has a reclining seat, you can begin using it while baby is still bottle feeding. As baby grows and sits up, you can adjust the highchair to a more upright position. A highchair brings your baby into the social scene of family meals. Even if the baby has already been fed, joining the family at mealtimes is a healthy, stimulating part of her day. Many highchairs are adaptable to a wide range of ages, which allows parents to transform these products from a highchair, to a safe resting place for a young infant, to a youth chair. Highchairs with this much versatility will take your child from infancy through toddlerhood.

FEATURES TO LOOK FOR

✔ Overall Size

If space is a concern, many combination plastic and aluminum highchair models fold flat for storage. These chairs should always have a locking mechanism to prevent collapse while your baby is in them.

✔ Wide Base for Stability

A highchair constructed with a wide leg base is harder to tip over than one with a narrower base. The broader leg base also makes the chair easier to clean. If you select a highchair with wheels or casters, be sure they have brakes to hold the chair securely in place when it's in use.

✔ Comfort

The seat should be well padded. If the seat is upholstered, be sure the padding is thick and won't puncture easily. Make sure seams have no sharp edges to scratch baby's legs. If the upholstery has buttons, check for secure attachment. Feeding time can be messy, so you'll want padding and covers that you can remove and either wipe clean or machine wash.

✔ Reclining Seat

A reclining seat makes feeding time more comfortable for everyone, and it can also greatly enhance the chair's versatility. A highchair with a reclining seat can be great for a very young or sleepy baby, and it may be more comfortable than a fully upright seat when baby is drinking.

✔ Adjustability

A high chair with height adjustments can accommodate parents and tables of varying heights. If you're in the family room watching TV, you might want to lower the highchair so you can feed baby while you're sitting on the couch. If you're cooking in the kitchen, you will want to raise the highchair so you can feed baby from a standing position. And you can put the highchair at midlevel when baby joins you at the dinner table.

✔ Adjustable Tray

A good highchair tray should let you operate it with one hand while you're hold-ing the baby with the other. The tray should adjust to several different posi-tions and lock securely into place to accommodate your growing baby. Check the underside of the tray for holes or sharp edges that could cut or trap little fingers. Wraparound trays are great for keeping food and toys on the tray top. A high rim on the tray will contain spills. A tray that directs spills toward the front will keep your baby drier. Some of the newer highchairs have two trays: a dinner tray and regular tray. After baby is finished eating, pop off the dinner tray and put it in the dishwasher. Your baby can still sit and play at the regular tray while you finish your meal.

✔ Restraining System

Highchairs should have a five-point safety harness. The seat belts and crotch straps should be independent of the tray, and they should be constructed of a strong, durable fabric that "hugs" your baby into the seat. The seat belts should secure your baby firmly across the hips and between the legs to prevent him from standing up in the chair or slipping out from under the tray. The most effective straps and belts attach securely to the seat or to the lower part of the back of the chair. These items should be adjustable to accommodate your growing child. The safety buckle should be absolutely foolproof. For example, a latch that is shallow or simple to operate can easily be undone, even by the pressure of baby's big tummy. And be sure to always use the restraining straps to protect your child from serious injury.

✔ Locking Device

Be certain the locking device works easily and properly to prevent the chair from accidentally folding. Make sure that wheeled highchairs have a tight lock-ing mechanism to prevent accidental rolling. If you'll be folding the chair after each use, test a number of chairs for easy operation. If space is an issue, you'll want the high chair to fold compactly and stand upright when folded.

✔ Easy Cleaning
Baby food has a way of getting into every nook and cranny of the highchair.
Check the seat, harness, tray, and frame for tiny, hard-to-wipe areas. Any fabrics should be plastic or vinyl so you can easily wipe them clean; dark fabrics
tend to camouflage stubborn stains. Many highchairs come with removable,
machine-washable seat pads.

✔ Footrest
A footrest is a nice feature for older babies, especially if it adjusts to accommodate your baby's growth.

✔ Splinterproof
If the chair is wooden, make sure it has a smooth finish and is free of splinters.

✔ Assembly
Some highchairs are ready to use out of the box, while others require assembly. It might be worth paying a little extra for a preassembled model if you're
not mechanically inclined.

○ Standard Highchairs
As with all baby products, make sure the highchair you buy conforms to all
current safety standards. Look for the Juvenile Products Manufacturers Association (JPMA) approval sign on the box.

- Aquarium Healthy Care High Chair by Fisher Price
  Manufacturer Web site: www.fisher-price.com
  The Aquarium Healthy Care High Chair will keep baby entertained
  while you prepare dinner or clean up in the kitchen. The highchair
  comes with an interactive toy tray where baby can press a button to
  make aquarium fish swim, or to hear one of four ocean sound effects.
  Baby can also use the highchair's roller to make music play. When
  baby's ready, the highchair coverts to a booster seat.

- Harmony Highchair by Graco
  Manufacturer Web site: www.gracobaby.com
  The Harmony Highchair has a kitchen-themed toy bar, which is a great
  way to entertain your baby while you're getting meals ready. When it's
  time to eat, the toy bar conveniently rotates out of the way.

- Polly Highchair by Chicco
  Vendor Web sites: www.babies1st.com; www.babyuniverse.com; www
  .lullabyelane.com
  This highchair is top-of-the-line without the high-end price tag. It's
  ideal at mealtime and playtime, and the reclining seat makes it a great
  place for short naps.

- Prima Pappa Diner by Peg Perego
  Manufacturer Web site: www.perego.com

This top-quality highchair provides the ultimate eating environment for infants and toddlers and the most convenience. This pre-assembled highchair has the style and colors to coordinate nicely with any décor.

○ Highchair Accessories
These accessories include an extra food tray, activity tray, a strap to keep baby's toys and teethers close at hand, and a floor mat to protect your floors and carpets from spills.

● High Chair Activity Tray by Peg Perego
Manufacturer Web site: *www.perego.com*
The High Chair Activity Tray provides great entertainment for your baby while he's sitting in the highchair waiting to eat or playing while you're busy in the kitchen. The activity tray is designed to be mounted on the Prima Pappa and Roller highchairs.

● No Mess Mat by Munchkin
Manufacturer Web site: *www.munchkininc.com*
Large, 50-inch vinyl mats protect floors, tabletops, and furniture from spills, splatters, and all kinds of stains. The mats wipe clean with a damp cloth. They come in four fun characters—Dora the Explorer, Spongebob Squarepants, Lion, and Monkey.

● Prima Pappa Dinner Tray by Peg Perego
Vendor Web sites: *www.amazon.com*; *www.babyuniverse.com*
If you buy a used Prima Pappa or Roller (also by Peg Perego) highchair, or your original tray is getting worn out and you need a new tray, the Prima Pappa Dinner Tray is the perfect solution. The children's food tray can be mounted on the Prima Pappa and Roller highchairs.

● Secure-a-Toy by Baby Buddy
Manufacturer Web site: *www.babybuddy.com*
Secure-a-Toy keeps baby's favorite toys and teethers close at hand to prevent them from being dropped or misplaced.

● Sesame Street Meal & Play Mat by The First Years
Vendor Web sites: *www.babiesrus.com*; *www.babyant.com*; *www.baby universe.com*
The Sesame Street Meal & Play Mat covers your floor underneath baby's highchair to keep messes from ruining your carpet or floor.

My daughter just loves looking at the colorful pictures of Big Bird and Cookie Monster. Also, the Meal & Play Mat covers a large area and is very easy to clean—Holly

○ Portable Hook-On Highchairs

Some parents prefer to get a portable highchair rather than a standard one. Portable hook-on highchairs attach easily to standard tables. These chairs take up less room, are great for traveling, and cost less than standard high-chairs. A portable highchair should have a safety strap and crotch strap for maximum security. The chair should have a high backrest and rigid seat for baby's comfort and support. A removable and washable fabric cover with a back storage pocket also is a nice feature. The chair seat should fold for travel. When you're using a hook-on chair, never place the chair where the child can push off with his feet and dislodge the chair.

- Fast Table Chair by Inglesina
  Manufacturer Web site: *www.inglesina.com*

- Hippo Hook-On Chair by Chicco
  Vendor Web sites: *www.babiesrus.com; www.babystyle.com; www.baby universe.com*

○ Portable Booster Seats

Like the portable hook-on highchairs, booster seats are great if you are short of kitchen space, and for eating on the go. Look for a booster seat that will grow with your baby from infancy through the toddler stages. The booster seat should have a reclining feature and adjustable height levels that let you feed your baby at the appropriate angle for her stage of development. The seat should have a three-point safety restraint with an easy-release buckle.

- Reclining Feeding Seat by The First Years
  Vendor Web sites: *www.babyant.com; www.babyuniverse.com; www.lullaby lane.com*
  Designed for infants and toddlers, this great space-saving alternative to a highchair includes a full-size pad for baby's comfort and a reversible tray mat that makes mealtime educational and fun.

- Deluxe Recline & Grow 5 Stage Feeding Seat by Safety 1st
  Manufacturer Web site: *www.safety1st.com*
  The Deluxe Recline & Grow 5 Stage Feeding Seat can be reclined to accommodate an infant, adjusted upright to accommodate an older child, and can be used as a restaurant-style booster seat with no back-rest for toddlers.

○ Inflatable Portable Booster Seat

An inflatable portable booster seat is compact and lightweight, so you can take it anywhere you go. This option is perfect for restaurant dining.

- On-the-Go Booster Seat by The First Years
  Manufacturer Web site: *www.thefirstyears.com*
  The On-the-Go Booster Seat is great for traveling. When you want to use the seat just pull out the valve, and it self-inflates into a sturdy and comfortable full-size booster seat. The adjustable safety belt with

T-restraint helps hold your child in the seat. When mealtime is over, press out the air and fold down. For babies nine to thirty-six months.

Playards are versatile pieces of equipment. A playard is an enclosed space that gives your baby a place to play or nap. There are three types: basic playards, bassinet playards, and playpens. Basic playards double as a playpen and a crib for naps. The mattress lies at the bottom of the playard. Bassinet playards have a built-in bassinet for newborns. The bassinets are designed to hold newborns up until they weigh 15 pounds. When your baby outgrows the bassinet, simply remove it to create a sleeping or play area. A changing station might be a feature that comes with your playard, or you can purchase it separately if your playard does not include one. The changing station provides a convenient, safe, and sanitary place to change your baby.

FEATURES TO LOOK FOR

✔ Sturdy but Lightweight
You will probably be moving the playard around a lot, so you want one that's lightweight and well built.

✔ Narrow Width
If you plan to move your playard from room to room, it should be narrow enough to fit through doorways.

✔ Wheels
For easy maneuverability, the playard should have two wheels that lock for safety.

✔ See-Through Mesh Netting Around the Sides
The mesh netting lets you keep an eye on your baby and your baby see what's going on around him.

✔ Bassinet
A bassinet elevates baby to a higher level in the Pack 'n Play. This makes it easier to care for baby when he's not sleeping.

✔ Changing Table
A changing table makes it convenient to change baby right in the playard, especially if the playard is set up in a room other than the nursery.

✔ Canopy
If you plan to use your playard outdoors, look for one that has a canopy, which protects baby from the sun's UV rays and provides shade to keep him cooler.

✔ Netting
Netting protects your baby from mosquitoes and other insects.

✔ Easy Push-Button Fold
Because playards are frequently used for traveling, they should fold down easily and compactly.

EXTRA FEATURES

✔ Vibration system—soothes and lulls your baby to sleep.

✔ Mobile—helps little eyes focus on objects.

✔ Attached soft toys—makes the playard more fun.

✔ Music—lets you play soothing lullabies and classical tunes.

✔ Night Light—lets you check on your baby without waking him up.

✔ Toy Bag—nice to have to store all those extra playthings or supplies.

○ Pack 'n Play Playards
If you want your newborn to sleep in your room for awhile, you can use a bassinet playard instead of setting up a full-size crib. If you have a two-story house, put the full-size crib upstairs in the nursery for nighttime, and set up a playard downstairs to use during the day. This arrangement saves you from having to run up and down the stairs all day long when baby needs you. Playards are a safe place for baby to sleep or play when they're visiting Grandma or going for an outing to the park or beach.

● Contours 2-in-1 Travel Playard by Kolcraft
Manufacturer Web site: *www.kolcraft.com*
This is a versatile playard with music, vibrations, soft toy mobile, removable bassinet, and soft parent organizer. The Soft-Glow Check Light with one-minute timer lets you check your baby at night.

● Jeep Sahara Limited XT by Kolcraft
Manufacturer Web site: *www.kolcraft.com*
This Pack 'n Play is the perfect choice for families who like to spend time outdoors, whether at the beach, the park, or in their own backyard. The roll-down weather screen and removable sunshade canopy protect your baby from the elements.

● Pack 'n Play Playards by Graco
Manufacturer Web site: *www.gracobaby.com*
There are so many Pack 'n Play models to choose from. A Pack 'n Play is perfect for staying at home or traveling. Take the convenience of a nursery with you wherever you and your little one go. Most units come complete with full-size bassinet and changing table. They also include battery-operated gentle vibrations and tranquil lullaby music, both of which come with timers so they turn off automatically.

● Twins Bassinet Playard by Graco
Manufacture Web site: *www.gracobaby.com*
The Twins Bassinet portable playard features a double bassinet for twins. The bassinets are lined with Graco's signature quilted bumper and mattress pads for added comfort. Dual canopies block lights for naptime.

○ Pack 'n Play Accessories

These products will accessorize your Pack 'N Play playard. Having a canopy, netting, electronic vibrating system, or cabana kit will make your Pack 'N Play a more comfortable place for baby to nap or play. And keeping extra pads, sheets, and a diaper organizer handy will make the playard more convenient for you.

- Pack 'n Play Changing Table Pad Covers by Graco
  Manufacturer Web site: *www.gracobaby.com*
  This changing pad cover is a great solution to avoid putting baby down on a cold surface, and it keeps the changing pad clean.

- Pack 'n Play Playard Diaper Organizer by Graco
  Vendor Web site: *www.babies1st.com*
  The diaper organizer keeps all of your diaper-changing essentials within reach. You can keep lotion and diaper-rash ointments in the mesh pockets, and up to twelve diapers in the removable diaper stacker. A covered wipes case prevents wipes from drying out.

- Pack 'n Play Netting
  Vendor Web sites: *www.babyage.com*; *www.kidsurplus.com*
  This netting completely covers the playard's mesh sides to keep all insects and mosquitoes away from baby.

- Pack 'n Play Pad by Colgate (search by brand)
  Vendor Web site: *www.babycatalog.com*
  If you need to replace your Pack 'n Play pad, you will know where to find one.

Our son slept in his Pack 'N Play, right by our bed, for the first three months. He especially seemed to like the classical songs on it. The vibrating bassinet put him right to sleep.—Joann

- Pack 'n Play Sheets by Graco
  Manufacturer Web site: *www.gracobaby.com*
  You should purchase sheets specifically made for playards separately if you intend to use your playard as a crib for naps. The sheets will keep the playard clean, and your baby comfortable.

- Pack 'n Play Twins Playard Sheets
  Manufacturer Web site: *www.gracobaby.com*
  These sheets are made specially for the Twins Bassinet Playard

- Pack 'n Play Playard Electronics Unit
  Manufacturer Web site: *www.gracobaby.com*

This unit will soothe and entertain your baby with its five classical songs, five soothing nature sounds, and a soft illuminating night light. With four timer settings you can choose the soothing time that fits your baby's needs.

- Portable Playard Tent plus Cabana Kit by Tots in Mind

  Manufacturer Web site: *www.totsinmind.com*

  This protective playard tent protects against climbing accidents, thrown toys, and unwanted pet visitors.

○ Traditional Square Playpens

You can keep your baby safe and secure in a traditional playpen while you're busy doing things around the house. If you are looking for a playard that looks like an old-fashioned square playpen, here are some suggestions.

- Li'l Playzone with Lights & Sounds by One Step Ahead

  Manufacturer Web site: *www.onestepahead.com*

  This expandable playard entertains with lights and sounds. The playard assembles quickly into various configurations, then breaks down into portable, easy-to-store pieces. The playard's wall of toys keeps your child amused, with a telephone, mirror, bead rollers, and a new keyboard that plays music and has flashing lights. This unit provides 13 square feet of space, or you can enlarge it by adding up to five extensions. The playard has a two-way door and a childproof lock.

We wanted a traditional square playpen. The Li'l Playzone is perfect. Our eight-month-old loves it. Its wall of toys with lights and sounds keeps him entertained for hours. —Molly

- Totblock by Graco

  Vendor Web sites: *www.babycatalog.com*; *www.babycenter.com*; *www.babyuniverse.com*

  This Pack 'N Play unit is two products in one: a playpen and a toy gym. The brightly colored, fun toys on the four mesh sides and the crisscross toy bar with more toys attached will be a source of amusement for your baby. The playmat is removable. You can place the playmat on the floor and attach the toy bar, and you have a toy gym to entertain baby. The push-button fold mechanism makes setting up and taking down this unit easy. The Totblock is perfect for play at home or on the go.

A stroller is an essential piece of baby gear. You cannot carry your child around on your hip for the next three years. Yet choosing the right stroller seems to be one of the biggest dilemmas expectant parents face. With all the types, brands, and models of strollers on the market, it's easy to feel overwhelmed. How do you know which stroller is right for you? Do you want a lightweight stroller, a standard stroller, a travel system, an old-fashioned carriage stroller, a jogging stroller, a "Snap-N-Go" stroller, or an umbrella stroller? If you are having multiples you will have to decide between a side-by-side stroller and a tandem stroller. With all these choices, you see how confusion can set in. Selecting a stroller is a personal decision. We are all looking for features that fit our own daily needs. With a little patience and research, you can find the right stroller for your lifestyle and budget.

If you can, when you're ready to buy a stroller, go to your local baby store and take a look at the strollers that interest you the most—the ones that you think have the features you're looking for. Give them a test run. Push them up and down aisles and through doorways to see how they maneuver. See how easy they are to open and fold. Practice putting them in and taking them out of your car. Doing all these things should make it easier for you to decide which stroller will be best for you and your family.

FEATURES TO LOOK FOR

✔ Seat Belts

Look for a five-point harness. The five-point harness has shoulder straps and will keep even the most rambunctious child in the seat. The buckle should be easy for you to undo, yet comfortable for your child.

✔ Multi-Position Reclining Seat

A fully reclining seat is a must for newborns.

✔ Adjustable Handle Height

Make sure the stroller fits you. Some strollers have handles with one fixed position. Others have height adjustments that might be easier on your back. Some handles are reversible so smaller infants can face you while you're pushing rather than looking out at what is in front of the stroller. Padded and ergonomically designed handles offer additional comfort for Mom and Dad. The ideal handle height is waist level or slightly below. Most strollers are built for the average-sized woman. If you don't fit this description (and most dads don't), you will want a stroller with adjustable handlebars.

✔ Canopy

An adjustable canopy will protect your child from the sun, rain, and wind. Some strollers have a viewing window in the canopy so you can see your baby at all times.

✔ **Storage Basket**
A storage basket is a necessity. Consider the capacity and accessibility of storage options when you are purchasing your stroller. The basket is great for carrying baby's essentials and for storing all those packages when you go on shopping sprees.

✔ **Footrest**
A footrest gives your baby a place to put his feet while you're going on a stroll.

✔ **Thick Padding**
Thick padding makes for a more comfortable ride.

✔ **Removable, Washable Fabric**
Wherever your baby goes, messy spills and crumbs are sure to follow. Whatever the seating type, removable, machine-washable padding and covers make cleanup easier.

✔ **Easy Handling**
As mentioned previously, test the stroller's maneuverability. You should be able to push the stroller in a straight line and turn it with one hand. These capabilities let you open and go through doorways easily and carry objects in the other hand.

✔ **One-Handed Folding Mechanism**
A stroller should fold and unfold with ease. Some strollers employ automatic locks for hassle-free handling. As mentioned previously, open and close the stroller in the store, and make sure you are comfortable with its operation before you make the purchase.

✔ **Wheel Types**
Front and rear swivel wheels make a stroller easier to move, while wheels that move only in one position generally handle more awkwardly. Unless you're looking for the additional stability offered by fixed-position and oversized wheels, which you'll usually find on sport models, fully independent wheels are recommended for mall and supermarket use. Their caster-like movement allows for the best maneuverability, and many models feature a locking device to point the front wheels straight ahead for added stability.

✔ **Brakes**
Test the brakes in the store. Make sure they are easy to operate. The wheels should lock when you engage the brake. Two braking wheels are preferable to only one for holding the stroller securely.

✔ **Security**
Make sure your stroller has an easy-to-use locking mechanism that prevents it from collapsing accidentally.

Stroller Safety

Safety should be the top priority when you're buying a stroller. No matter what the brand name or price of the stroller, if it doesn't provide the ultimate in safety, the name and price mean nothing. Being informed is your best protection when you're choosing and using a stroller. All strollers are not equally safe. The majority of strollers on the market today pass the strict Juvenile Product Manufacturers Association (JPMA) rigorous safety standards. The JPMA tests products for, among other things, secure restraint systems, protection against unexpected tipping, and safety from loose parts that might present a choking hazard. Look for safety-certified strollers, or call the JPMA at 1-609-231-8500 for a list of certified strollers.

SAFETY FEATURES

✔ Wide Base

A stroller or carriage with a wide base will prevent tipping. When your baby leans over the side, the stroller should remain erect.

✔ Tipping Backward

The stroller should resist tipping backward when you press downward lightly on the handle. When the seat adjusts to a reclining position, make sure the stroller doesn't tip backward when the child lies down. Don't hang your purse, diaper bag, or shopping bags over the handles. If your stroller has a shopping basket for carrying packages, the basket should be low on the back of the stroller or directly over the rear wheels.

✔ Sharp Edges or Gaps

Check the stroller frame for hazardous sharp edges or gaps that could injure a child's small fingers or toes. Avoid safety-bar openings or leg holes wide enough for an infant to accidentally slip through. Be sure plastic end caps on tube ends are fastened securely.

✔ Canopy Window

A model that lets you keep an eye on your baby while you're strolling might give you a little extra peace of mind.

✔ Pillow

Never use a pillow in a stroller for an infant.

✔ Safety Harness

Always secure baby by using the restraint system.

✔ Brakes

Apply the brakes to limit rotation of the wheels when the stroller is stationary. Never rely on a stroller's brakes alone to secure your baby on an inclined surface.

✔ Locking Device

Use the locking device to prevent accidental folding.

✔ Folding Strollers

Select a stroller that opens and closes easily. If you are alone with your child, a stroller with a one-hand fold mechanism is ideal. Keep children away when you are folding and unfolding a stroller. To keep your stroller in top-notch safety condition, give it a frequent checkup. Tighten nuts and bolts, replace worn straps, examine the brakes, and lubricate the wheels.

✔ Weight and Maneuverability
When you're shopping for a double or triple stroller, consider the weight and manageability of various models. Try before you buy.

✔ Not a Toy
Don't let children use a stroller as a toy.

✔ Child Safety
Never leave a child unattended in a stroller.

✔ Stairs and Escalators
Never attempt to carry your baby in the stroller, especially on stairs and escalators.

✔ Weight Capacity
Strollers should be used only for children who weigh up to 35 or 40 pounds.

Strollers for a Single Baby

So where should you begin to decide what stroller style would be right for your family? There are so many different models to choose from. The first thing to consider is your lifestyle. Before you buy a stroller, consider where you live, where you plan to push your stroller, and how much you want to spend. If you live in a city and plan to take your child on urban hikes, you'll need a stroller that's sturdy but easy to maneuver up curbs and in and out of shops and narrow aisles. If you're a suburban parent who uses a stroller mainly for quick trips to the store, you can probably get away with something lighter and cheaper. Active moms and dads who hope to take their baby on jogs or hikes in rough terrain will want to buy a rugged jogging stroller. Parents who travel frequently will need a lightweight stroller that folds up compactly so it's easy to carry on a plane or wherever they go. Listed are various types of strollers. Select a stroller that you feel would be most appropriate for your style of living.

○ Umbrella Strollers
Umbrella strollers are so named because they fold up similar to an umbrella. These models are usually the most compact and inexpensive. Umbrella strollers offer few comfort features, but they are the most convenient. The umbrella stroller is great when you have to take your child with you to do errands, and you will be getting in and out of the car frequently. This style is lightweight and folds easily. If you have multiples, you can buy two lightweight umbrella strollers and put them together with a stroller connector to make one side-by-side multiple stroller. If Mom and Dad want to go their separate ways with one baby each, they have two single umbrella strollers at hand. An umbrella stroller is recommended for children who are old enough to hold their heads up on their own.

- Caddy Stroller by Chicco
  Vendor Web sites: *www.babyuniverse.com*; *www.dreamtimebaby.com*; *www.target.com*
  The Chicco Caddy Stroller is a great little stroller at a great price. The simplest of umbrella strollers, this is the perfect stroller to leave at Grandma's house or take traveling. It has many of the features and amenities you would expect to find on a full-size stroller. This stroller weighs 11 pounds.

- Tour Sport Reclining Umbrella Stroller by Kolcraft
  Manufacturer Web site: *www.kolcraft.com*
  The Kolcraft Reclining Umbrella Stroller is thoughtfully designed and carefully constructed with your baby's comfort and safety in mind. This single umbrella stroller has the added feature of a semireclining padded seat not often found on lightweight umbrella strollers. This stroller weighs 11.22 pounds.

- Tour Sport Universal Reclining Umbrella Stroller by Kolcraft (new product)
  Manufacturer Web site: *www.kolcraft.com*
  The Tour Sport Universal Reclining Umbrella Stroller has all the amenities of a full-size stroller without the size, weight, or cost. The seat has a three-point harness and a multiposition reclining seat. The stroller has a spacious storage basket, a canopy with a top window, and a cup holder. The stroller accommodates most infant car seats and delivers comfort and convenience at a great price. It weighs 12 pounds.

- Volo by Maclaren
  Manufacturer Web site: *www.maclarenbaby.com*
  Volo answers the needs of busy families on the go. Its stunningly simple design meets the practical demands of travel and portability. The stroller has a removable canopy and a removable mesh storage basket. The convenient shoulder strap makes it easy to transport wherever you go. This stroller weighs 9.2 pounds.

○ Lightweight Strollers
Lightweight strollers usually weigh 12 pounds or less. These strollers are ideal for travel, quick trips to the store, or for those parents for whom lifting poses a problem. Lightweight strollers are designed for easy maneuverability, and the best of them have many excellent features, such as thick padding, adjustable sun canopies, cup holders, and easy-to-operate brakes. They fold quickly and easily, and some even stash into overhead compartments on planes. If your lightweight stroller fully reclines, you can use it with your newborn. Otherwise, wait to use it until your child is four to six months old.

- Aria OH Stroller by Peg Perego
  Manufacturer Web site: *www.perego.com*

This lightweight stroller is perfect for quick trips or for traveling. It has everything you want in a convenience stroller, and it is extremely durable as well. This stroller can also serve as a travel system, thanks to the retractable car-seat anchors that instantly attach a Primo Viaggio infant car seat to the stroller. The stroller weighs 10 pounds.

I have a bad back so I needed a lightweight stroller that would be easy to lift in and out of the car. The Aria is perfect! It steers easily, goes over bumps smoothly, and folds/opens in a snap.—Danielle

- City Savvy by Combi
  Manufacturer Web site: *www.combistrollers.com*
  The City Savvy is a must for parents on the go. The deep reclining seat accommodates an infant. Use the City Savvy by itself or combine it with the new Combi Connections car seat for a travel system that's only 17 pounds. The stroller by itself weighs 12 pounds.

○ Standard-Size Strollers
  Standard strollers are designed for more active parents who need a stroller that can stand up to more than shopping-mall conditions. Standard strollers are bigger and sturdier, but they're also heavier and more expensive than lightweight strollers. Standard strollers are designed for comfort and durability, so they're perfect if you plan on many long walks with baby. Most models feature fully reclining seats, which means they angle back to 170 degrees, making them suitable for newborns. Many models accept an infant car/seat carrier.

- Bugaboo Stroller—Gecko or Cameleon by Bugaboo
  Manufacture Web site: *www.bugaboostrollers.com*
  Bugaboo strollers are remarkably rugged, versatile strollers. They navigate superbly on either a city sidewalk or a bumpy hike in the woods. The Bugaboo has a strong yet lightweight aluminum chassis. Both a reversible, three-position recline seat for children up to 40 pounds, and an optional bassinet for newborns up to six months old or 19 pounds are included. For added convenience, the Graco SnugRide, Graco Infant Safe Seat (Step 1), or Peg Perego Primo Viaggio infant car seats can also be attached directly to the Bugaboo's base with special car-seat connectors. The stroller weighs 18 pounds.

- Combi I-Thru Stroller
  Manufacturer Web site: *www.combistrollers.com*

Combi's I-Thru Stroller features a stroller seat that detaches from the stroller frame so that the baby can look out at the world or be facing the parent. The I-Thru is a full-recline stroller with a full-size canopy. This stroller easily converts from a forward-facing to a bassinet-style stroller for newborns. The stroller weighs 16 pounds.

- MetroLite LE by Graco
  Manufacturer Web site: *www.gracobaby.com*
  A great stroller with all the features parents want, the lightweight aluminum frame of the MetroLite LE makes getting around a breeze. The never-flat rubber tires promise a smooth ride, and because they are made of solid rubber, they are puncture proof, so you should never have a flat tire. This stroller is compatible with the Graco SnugRide infant car seat. The stroller weighs 18 pounds.

- Pliko P3 Classico by Peg Perego
  Manufacturer Web site: *www.perego.com*
  This stroller has beautiful European styling and all the features for on-the-go families. Your baby can ride in the reclined seat or in a Primo Viaggio infant car seat. The stroller even has a rear footrest with a non-skid rubber insert for an older sibling or friend. The stroller weighs 15 pounds.

- Quattro Tour LXI by Graco
  Manufacturer Web site: *www.gracobaby.com*
  Designed with bike-frame technology, this aluminum stroller will give you years of comfy strolling for infants through toddlers. When folded, the stroller rests on the wheels so that it never comes in direct contact with the ground, which helps keep it clean. The Quattro Tour LXI is compatible with the Graco SnugRide infant car seat. This stroller weighs 25 pounds.

- Techno XT by Maclaren
  Manufacturer Web site: *www.maclarenbaby.com*
  The Techno XT is an all-terrain stroller with a sleek, sporty look and superior performance. You can use this stroller for newborns through toddlers. The stroller weighs 17 pounds.

○ Travel Systems
  Travel systems are strollers on which you snap an infant car seat. They are a multiuse product that accommodates a growing baby. They let you transport your baby without waking her after a car ride, a feature that parents love. The infant car seat can be used for infants up to 22 pounds and can also be used as a rocking carrier. As the child grows, you can use the stroller without the car seat. This category of products is both economical and extremely convenient.

  - Combi DK-5 Ultra Light Travel System
    Manufacturer Web site: *www.combistrollers.com*

The DK-5 Travel System is a lightweight and portable lifestyle travel system with state-of-the-art features! The energy-absorbing, patented Egg Shock foam in the stroller and Combi Connection infant seat offers uncompromising protection for your baby. Parents love the convenient one-hand, effortless open and fold. The infant boot keeps baby nice and warm in cold weather. This travel system weighs 21 pounds with a car-seat stroller included.

- MetroLite Travel System by Graco
  Manufacturer Web site: *www.gracobaby.com*
  This system offers comfort and on-the-go convenience at a great price. The travel system includes the LiteRider stroller, a SnugRide infant car seat, and a stay-in-car adjustable base. The stroller weighs 23 pounds

- Quattro Tour Travel System by Graco
  Manufacturer Web site: *www.gracobaby.com*
  The Quattro Tour Travel System is becoming popular with moms and dads everywhere. The three-piece set includes a Quattro Tour stroller, a SnugRide infant car seat, and a stay-in-car base. Designed with bike-frame technology, this aluminum stroller promises years of comfy strolling for infants through toddlers. When folded, the stroller rests on the wheels so that it never comes in contact with the ground, which helps keep it clean. This stroller weighs 27 pounds.

○ Snap-N-Go Strollers
  Snap-N-Go strollers are a wonderful invention. Now you can transfer your infant car seat/carrier to a stroller frame without disturbing your baby. A Snap-N-Go stroller is an extremely lightweight, compact metal frame into which you snap the infant car seat. It is the perfect antidote to bulky travel systems. The Snap-N-Go strollers feature a removable parent tray with dual cup holders, an extra-large storage basket, and convenient one-hand fold that lets you hold your child and fold the carrier at the same time. You can use a Snap-N-Go stroller frame only until your baby outgrows the infant car seat.

  - Snap N Go by Baby Trend
    Manufacturer Web site: *www.babytrend.com*
    The Snap N Go accommodates most Century, Evenflo, Graco, Cosco, and Gerry infant car seats. It folds easily and can fit in an overhead compartment on an airplane. The stroller frame weighs 11 pounds.

  - SnugRider Stroller by Graco
    Manufacturer Web site: *www.gracobaby.com*
    The SnugRider Stroller is engineered exclusively for the SnugRide Infant Car Seat. This lightweight stroller frame weighs only 12 pounds, making it the perfect portable accessory for your Graco Infant Car Seat.

  - Universal Car Seat Carrier by Kolcraft
    Manufacturer Web site: *www.kolcraft.com*

The Universal Car Seat Carrier accommodates Britax, Century, Combi, Cosco, Evenflo, Graco, and Safety 1st car seats. The stroller frame weighs 13.5 pounds.

○ Jogging Strollers

Jogging strollers are an ideal solution for people who want and need to weave exercise into their new lives as parents. Jogging strollers feature three large, shock-absorbent bicycle wheels mounted to a lightweight frame. These strollers can handle all types of terrain, including grass, sand, gravel, and so on. The thick rubber wheels make for a smooth ride just about anywhere. Jogging strollers are great for taking your child on long walks, runs, hikes, and even walks through the shopping mall. Note that many pediatricians recommend not running with your baby in a jogger stroller until she is six months old, or until she can hold her head up on her own.

- Baby Jogger Performance Series by Baby Jogger
  Manufacturer Web site: *www.babyjogger.com*
  This stroller is extremely lightweight and easy to push. The very best stroller for hard-core running, it has many great features, such as built-in shock absorbers and an updated sun canopy. This stroller weighs 16.5 pounds.

- Ironman Stroller by BOB
  Manufacturer Web site: *www.bobstrollers.com*
  The Ironman strollers are the lightest of the BOB line. These strollers are made for parents who love to run and want to bring their child along for the ride. The high-quality slick tires minimize rolling resistance, while the stiffer suspension maximizes maneuverability and response. The Ironman is versatile and portable, so it can easily be packed into a car and serve all your stroller needs. The stroller weighs 20 pounds.

- Jeep Overland Limited Jogging Stroller by Kolcraft
  Manufacturer Web site: *www.kolcraft.com*
  Now you and your child can listen to music as you jog along. The Music on the Move Parent Tray allows parent and baby to enjoy their favorite tunes using their own CD or MP3 player. The stroller includes speakers, an amplifier, and a source for output. This lightweight stroller has a height-adjustable Smart Handle so you can maintain good running form and posture. A trip odometer monitors speed and distance as you jog along.

- Revolution Stroller by BOB
  Manufacturer Web site: *www.bobstrollers.com*
  This stroller is truly the SUV of jogging strollers—it lets you give your baby a cushy ride on easygoing walks or serious runs over the roughest terrain. The stroller weighs 22.5 pounds.

○ Car Seat Adapter for Jogging Stroller
  ● Infant Car Seat Adapter by BOB
    Manufacturer Web site: *www.bobstrollers.com*
    This accessory allows for use of popular infant car seat models with BOB's single-seat jogging strollers.

○ Carriages and Prams
  A carriage or pram is the most elegant mode for promenading baby. Carriages and prams are especially suitable for newborns because they offer a fully reclining sleep space, extra cushioning, and big chrome wheels that deliver a super-smooth ride. Some carriages and prams convert from a fully horizontal riding position to an upright sitting position, like other types of strollers do. You'll pay more for carriages or prams, and they're not as portable, but many of them are heirloom-quality purchases that can be passed down and cherished for generations. Some carriages come with separate bassinets, giving you two great baby habitats in one. Urban parents especially appreciate the carriage because it offers such excellent protection from the elements and looks so stylish.
  ● Carriages and Prams by Inglesina
    Manufacturer Web site: *www.inglesina.com*
    Inglesina's carriages and prams epitomize the quality, style, and fashionable appeal of trips to the park with baby in a buggy. The weight will depend on the size and style of the carriage or pram.
  ● Culla Carriage Stroller by Peg Perego
    Vendor Web sites: *www.babyuniverse.com*; *www.dealtime.com*
    This modular system comes complete with chassis, all-season bassinet, and luxurious stroller seat. The Primo Viaggio car seat instantly attaches directly onto the chassis. The bassinet includes an adjustable backrest and can be used off-chassis as a portable cradle.

○ Tandem Strollers with Stadium Seating
  The tandem stroller with stadium seating is great for a family with an infant and a sibling. These strollers have one fully reclining seat that will accept an infant car-seat carrier. The other seat partially reclines. Stadium seating lets the child riding in the back have a good view of his surroundings.
  ● Jeep Wagoneer SE or Limited by Kolcraft
    Manufacturer Web site: *www.kolcraft.com*
    The Jeep Wagoneer is a rugged, good-looking stroller with a rear seat that will accommodate most infant car seats. A front-seat activity center with an electronic steering wheel will delight toddlers and older drivers. This stroller weighs 36.3 pounds.
  ● Take Me Too! Express Tandem Stroller by Evenflo
    Manufacturer Web site: *www.evenflo.com*

The Take Me Too! is a sturdy tandem stroller with versatile seating options. The MyStep side-entry provides easy in and out for toddlers and easy basket access for parents. The rear seat secures major brands of infant car seats to make a travel system.

- Express Rider Universal by Kolcraft
Manufacturer Web site: *www.kolcraft.com*
The Express Rider Universal is perfect for a family on the go! The rear seat will accommodate most brands of infant car seats. The stroller weighs 26 pounds.

Strollers for Multiples

If you're expecting your second child or multiples, your first consideration is how you want your children to ride. Do you want a side-by-side, tandem, or jogging stroller?

Twin Strollers

○ Twin Side-by-Side Strollers
The best side-by-side strollers are narrower than you think (only 30 inches wide), have independently reclining seats, and are suitable for babies from birth to 40 pounds. A side-by-side stroller with a handle that extends all the way across the back of the stroller is easier to control. A side-by-side stroller with umbrella handles is harder to maneuver. A side-by-side stroller makes it easy for you to tend to each baby when necessary. Two children communicate with each other in a side-by-side stroller, and each child has an equal view of the world. Many parents think a side-by-side stroller is best for twins because it solves the problem of who rides in front.

Our twins love riding in their side-by-side stroller. They can see each other, interact easily, and they each have an equal view of what's going on around them.—Monica

- Aria Twin by Peg Perego
Manufacturer Web site: *www.perego.com*
This is the ultimate convenience stroller for two children, and great for those quick trips or when traveling. The Aria Twin is amazingly light and comfortable. This stroller weighs 15 pounds.
- DuoRider by Graco
Manufacturer Web site: *www.gracobaby.com*

This basic double stroller is designed keeping in mind convenience for you and comfort for your babies. It is medium weight, easy to maneuver, and reasonably priced. The stroller weighs 23 pounds.

- Tour Mate Umbrella Stroller by Kolcraft
  Manufacturer Web site: *www.kolcraft.com*
  This simple, lightweight stroller is easy to transport, and it's perfect when both children want a front-seat view. Parents will love the gear bags and cup holder just for them. This stroller weighs 23.5 pounds.

- Twin Savvy EX by Combi
  Manufacturer Web site: *www.combistrollers.com*
  The Combi Acoustic Canopy strollers have miniature stereo speakers set in a pocket on either side of the canopy, so you can comfort your babies with soothing music, entertain them with fairytales, or educate them with the ABCs. The stroller weighs 21 pounds.

- Twin Techno by Maclaren
  Manufacturer Web site: *www.maclarenbaby.com*
  The Twin Techno is a great umbrella-style stroller. Moms appreciate the quick and easy Maclaren umbrella-style fold. The stroller weighs 25.7 pounds.

- Urban Double by Mountain Buggy
  Manufacturer Web site: *www.mountainbuggy.com*
  The Urban Double sets new standards for all-terrain double strollers. Only 29 inches wide, it will fit through a standard doorway and hold two passengers, from newborn through about four years of age. Turn this stroller into a pram with an optional CarryCot or twin bassinet. Bring along an older child by attaching an optional KiddyBoard. The stroller weighs 31 pounds.

○ Twin Tandem Strollers
Tandem strollers seat children one behind the other. The tandem car-seat combination strollers let you take your babies from the car to the stroller without waking them up. However, some parents feel that after adding the car seats, the stroller becomes a heavy piece of equipment and is harder to maneuver. Some parents also feel they don't use the car-seat attachment that often. For example, if you're taking the babies to the doctor or to visit family or friends, you usually don't take the whole stroller in with you, but take only the babies in the car seats. So before you buy a twin tandem stroller with attachable car seats, give it a test drive to make sure it won't be too heavy for you to maneuver once you add the babies.

- Duette SW by Peg Perego
  Manufacturer Web site: *www.perego.com*
  Elegant and roomy, this tandem stroller is the perfect choice for strolling two in style—it accommodates two infant car seats for a complete

travel system. The seats can be positioned to face front, rear, or each other. This stroller weighs 39.2 pounds.

- DuoGlider by Graco
  Manufacturer Web site: *www.gracobaby.com*
  The DuoGlider is a sturdy, attractive, and roomy double stroller that's compatible with Graco SnugRide infant car seats. When used with two infant car seats, the stroller transforms into a complete twin travel system. The stroller weighs 37 pounds.

- Sport Double Stroller by Runabout
  Vendor Web sites: *www.babies1st.com*; *www.comfortfirst.com*
  At only 24 inches wide, this stroller is easy to maneuver on sidewalks and jogging trails, through doorways, or in the mall. It's ideal for walking or jogging on all types of terrain.

○ Twin Jogging Strollers
  Like the single jogging strollers, twin jogging strollers are an ideal solution for new parents who want to weave exercise into their lives and take their kids along for the ride. As mentioned previously, be aware that many pediatricians recommend not running with your babies in a jogging stroller until they are six months old or until they can hold their heads up on their own

- Ironman Duallie by BOB
  Manufacturer Web site: *www.bobstrollers.com*
  With a smooth-riding jogging stroller for two, a growing family doesn't have to slow you down. The Ironman Sport Utility Stroller Duallie D'Lux includes stainless-steel spokes and aluminum wheels to reduce weight and improve handling and performance. This stroller weighs 28.9 pounds.

- Performance Series Double Stroller by Babyjogger
  Manufacturer Web site: *www.babyjogger.com*
  The side-by-side seating in this stroller works just great. This stroller is so well balanced that you can use it with one child or two, or two of the same or very different sizes. The stroller weighs 42 pounds.

- Run Around Double by Instep
  Manufacturer Web site: *www.instep.net*
  Double the fun on your walks or runs with this lightweight, easy-to-maneuver double jogging stroller. Busy parents can stay in shape and bring the little ones along. This indoor/outdoor jogger is at home on the sidewalk, in the park, and even in the mall. It's perfect for short runs or long walks. This stroller weighs 30 pounds.

Triplet Strollers

Taking three babies out at a time is no problem if you have the right stroller. If you like the idea of owning one stroller that will accommodate three children of the same or various ages, then one of the following recommended side-by-side, tandem, or jogging strollers might be for you.

- ○ Triplet Side-by-Side Stroller
  - • Urban Triple Jogging Stroller by Mountain Buggy
    Manufacturer Web site: *www.mountainbuggy.com*
    Rugged, versatile and convenient, the Urban Triple, with two swiveling front wheels that can easily be locked, sets new standards for all-terrain triple strollers The stroller is only 42 inches wide and will hold three passengers from newborn through about four years of age, or any combination in between. This stroller weighs 43 pounds.

- ○ Triplet Tandem Strollers
  - • Runabout Triple Stroller
    Vendor Web sites: *www.babies1st.com*; *www.tripletconnection.com*
    The Runabout stroller is lightweight and only 24 inches wide, so you can easily maneuver on sidewalks, through doorways, or in the mall. This stroller handles beautifully on all types of terrain. Take a walk on the beach, on jogging trails, on gravel roads, on light snow, or anywhere you want to go. Reclining seats and a telescoping handle make outings comfortable for parents and babies.
  - • Triplette SW by Peg Perego
    Manufacturer Web site: *www.perego.com*
    The Peg Perego Triplette SW Stroller is perfect for all three little passengers. This stroller features an instant G-matic seat attachment for two car seats. The stroller weighs 46 pounds.

- ○ Triplet Jogging Stroller
  - • Q Series Triple Jogging Stroller by Baby Jogger
    Manufacturer Web site: *www.babyjogger.com*
    This triple jogger is enjoyed by families all over the world. The stroller can be used for a set of triplets or three kids of different ages. The stroller is balanced so kids can sit in any seat they want to. Individual multiposition sun canopies with clear-view windows let you see all three babies at all times. The stroller features the new Quick Folding System—simply lift and fold for easy storage. The stroller weighs 44.5 pounds.

Quad Strollers

Do you need a stroller for four? If you're a parent of quads or you run a day-care center, then these are the strollers for you.

- ○ Quad Side-by-Side Strollers
  - • Bye-Bye Buggy—4 Seater by Backyard Adventures
    Manufacturer Web site: *www.byebyebuggy.com*

The Bye-Bye Buggy has terraced seats so all children have an equal view of the world. The front wheels pivot 360 degrees. Other features include a user-friendly safety brake and a built-in storage compartment. The canopy and infant seat are sold separately. This stroller accommodates children five months to thirty-six months of age. The stroller weighs 50 pounds.

- Quad Stroller
  Vendor Web sites: *www.daycaremall.com*; *www.showeryourbaby.com*
  This is a four-passenger commercial stroller with dual canopies that's great for parents of quads. The Quad Stroller is a sturdy stroller that features a runaway brake that engages when the grip handle is released, to let the person pushing it maintain control of the stroller. There are also ten large wheels for easy, smooth operation, as well as extra-large storage baskets. The stroller weighs 60 pounds.

○ Quad Tandem Stroller

- Runabout Quad 4 Seater Stroller
  Vendor Web sites: *www.babies1st.com*; *www.tripletconnection.com*
  Line your little ones up in this narrow, easy-to-maneuver tandem quad stroller and be on your way. The thin-wall steel, welded frame is light, solid, and glides along with ease. All Runabout Strollers are only 24 inches wide, so you can easily maneuver on sidewalks and jogging trails, through doorways, or in the mall.

Snap-N-Go Strollers

As mentioned previously, a Snap-N-Go stroller is an extremely light-weight, compact, metal frame into which you snap the infant car seat. This option is great for newborns and young babies. You can use the Snap-N-Go frame only until your baby outgrows the infant car seat.

○ Snap-N-Go Strollers for Multiples

- Double Decker Stroller For Twins and Triple Decker Stroller for Trip-lets by Doubledecker
  Manufacturer Web site: *www.doubledeckerstroller.com*
  The double-decker strollers for twins and the triple-decker strollers for triplets were invented by a mom and dad of multiples who know how difficult it is to be on the go with twins or triplets. These innova-tive stroller frames work with 3 Evenflo Discovery, On My Way, Cozy-Carry, PortAbout, or Graco SnugRide infant car seats.

- Double Snap N Go LX by Baby Trend
  Manufacturer Web site: *www.babytrend.com*
  This stroller offers a highly convenient way to transport two babies in their car seats—there's no need to disturb your babies during the transition from car to stroller. The stroller frame weighs 18 pounds.

Depending on the stroller you purchase, it might come with extra features, or it might not. The following list lets you know what products are available to make your stroller more comfortable and functional.

Stroller Weather Shields

Bad weather is no reason for you and your baby to stay inside. Stroller weather shields protect baby from wind, rain, and snow. These weather shields are durable, lightweight, and waterproof. They fit virtually any single or double stroller with a canopy. Netting on both sides allows for plenty of ventilation. Baby will stay dry and warm yet still be able to see out and enjoy the world. Carry the shields in your purse or stroller basket to be ready for those unpredictable weather changes.

- Single Stroller Rain Shields
  - Baby on Board Stroller Weather Shield by Safety 1st
    Manufacturer Web site: *www.safety1st.com*
  - Single Stroller Rain and Wind Cover by Protect-a-Bub
    Vendor Web sites: *www.babiesexpress.com*; *www.babyuniverse.com*
  - Small or Medium Rain Shield by Combi
    Manufacturer Web site: *www.combistrollers.com*
- Twin Side-by-Side Stroller Rain Shields
  - Side-by-Side Rain Cover by Protect-a-Bub
    Vendor Web sites: *www.babiesexpress.com*; *www.lullabylane.com*
- Twin Tandem Stroller Rain Shield
  - Duo Stroller Rain Cover by Graco
    Vendor Web sites: *www.babyuniverse.com*; *www.safeforbaby.com*
  - Tandem Rain Cover by Protect-a-Bub
    Vendor Web sites: *www.babiesexpress.com*; *www.lullabylane.com*
- Jogging Stroller Rain Shields
  - Double Weather Shield by BOB
    Manufacturer Web site: *www.bobstrollers.com*
  - Single Weather Shield by BOB
    Manufacturer Web site: *www.bobstrollers.com*
  - Twin Jogger Rain and Wind Cover by Protect-a-Bub
    Vendor Web sites: *www.babiesexpress.com*; *www.showeryourbaby.com*

Stroller Netting

Stroller netting keeps insects and mosquitoes away from your baby and protects your baby from 65 percent of harmful ultraviolet rays. Additionally, stroller netting shields baby against wind and dust, deters pets and strangers from touching your baby, and keeps your baby cooler in summer and warmer in winter.

- ○ Single-Stroller Netting
  - Baby on Board Stroller Netting by Safety 1st
    Manufacturer Web site: *www.safety1st.com*
  - BabyShade Adjustable Stroller Cover by Kiddopotamus
    Manufacturer Web site: *www.kiddopotamus.com*
  - Stroller Netting by Basic Comfort
    Vendor Web site: *www.babyabby.com*
- ○ Twin-Stroller Netting
  - Baby Shade Double Stroller Cover by Kiddopotamus
    Manufacturer Web site: *www.kiddopotamus.com*
  - Tandem Stroller Netting by Comfy Baby
    Vendor Web site: *www.babyage.com*
- ○ Single Jogging Stroller Netting
  - Sun and Wind Protector by BOB
    Manufacturer Web site: *www.bobstrollers.com*
- ○ Double Jogging Stroller Netting
  - Sun and Wind Protector by BOB
    Manufacturer Web site: *www.bobstrollers.com*

Sunshades

Protect your baby from the sun's harmful rays. Place the sunshades over any canopied stroller, jogger, or pram to provide protection in both sunny and overcast conditions. As the angle of the sun changes, you can adjust the canopy forward or back to give your child the right amount of sun protection.

- ○ Single-Stroller Sunshades
  - Jogger SunShade Attachment by Protect-a-Bub
    Vendor Web sites: *www.babies1st.com*; *www.babiesexpress.com*
  - RayShade UV Protective Stroller Sun Shade by Kiddopotamus
    Manufacturer Web site: *www.kiddopotamus.com*
  - Single Stroller Sunshade Attachment by Protect-a-Bub
    Vendor Web sites: *www.babyant.com*; *www.babiesexpress.com*
- ○ Double-Stroller Sun Shades
  - Double Wide RayShade by Kiddopotamus
    Manufacturer Web site: *www.kiddopotamus.com*
  - Twin Jogger Sunshade by Protect-a-Bub
    Vendor Web sites: *www.babiesexpress.com*; *www.target.com*
  - Twin Stroller Sunshade Attachment by Protect-a-Bub
    Vendor Web sites: *www.babiesexpress.com*; *www.babyuniverse.com*

Organizers, Holders, and Other Accessories

Stroller outings mean having a lot of extra baby necessities on hand. A wide range of options are available to help you organize and hold these many items, which just don't seem to all fit on the stroller itself. Other accessories, such as seat protectors, umbrellas, blankets, connectors, and extension handles, keep baby's stroller in top condition and make it more versatile as well.

○ Stroller Organizers
Sometimes the stroller basket is just not enough, especially if Mom is going shopping for herself. Stroller bags attach easily to the stroller handle to keep your baby's on-the-go essentials close at hand.

- Cup 'n Stuff Stroller Pocket by J. L. Childress
  Manufacturer Web site: *www.jlchildress.com*

- Stroller Bag by Prince Lionheart
  Manufacturer Web site: *www.princelionheart.com*

- Stroller Tote by J. L. Childress
  Manufacturer Web site: *www.jlchildress.com*

I use this on daily outings instead of a purse/diaper bag. It holds all of the essentials and leaves under the stroller free for other items. It easily snaps on and off for moving.—Mandy

○ Drink Holders
Drink holders conveniently attach to strollers to keep cups, cans, and baby bottles right at your fingertips.

- Click 'n Go Stroller Cup Holder by Prince Lionheart
  Manufacturer Web site: *www.princelionheart.com*

- Baby on Board Fold-Up Stroller Drink Holder by Safety 1st
  Manufacturer Web site: *www.safety1st.com*

- Stroll'r Hold'r II by Kel-Gar
  Manufacturer Web site: *www.kelgar.com*

○ Snack Holder
A hungry baby is a grumpy baby. Having snacks on hand can relieve a growling little tummy while you're out with baby. A snack holder attaches to the stroller so baby can eat merrily while you're strolling along.

- Click 'n Go Stroller Accessory System by Prince Lionheart
  Manufacturer Web site: *www.princelionheart.com*

○ Seat Protectors

Seat protectors make every seat accident proof. Protect your strollers, carriers, and car seats from leaking diapers, spilled food, and beverages. Cleanup is easy, and there will be no unsightly stains. Seat protectors also provide insulation and cushion baby's ride.

- Piddle Pad Waterproof Seat Liner by Kiddopotamus
  Manufacturer Web site: *www.kiddopotamus.com*
- StrollSoft Premium Seat Liner by Kiddopotamus
  Manufacturer Web site: *www.kiddopotamus.com*

○ Stroller Umbrellas

If your stroller doesn't have a canopy, the stroller umbrella is the perfect solution. Parents who enjoy taking their children out on warm, sunny days but are concerned about prolonged exposure to the heat and direct sun need not worry anymore. The umbrella provides shade right where baby needs it when you're outdoors. The umbrella is great for rainy days, too. These umbrellas attach to virtually all strollers, travel yards, back carriers, beach chairs, and wagons.

- Click 'n Go Stroller Umbrella by Prince Lionheart
  Vendor Web site: *www.kidsurplus.com*
- Infant Umbrella by Graco
  Vendor Web site: *www.babyage.com*

○ Stroller Blanket

Keep baby warm on cold days in a stroller blanket. The unique blanket-like design encloses kids' legs and keeps them warm even on windy days. The blanket attaches to any type of stroller—including jogging and double strollers—with Velcro fasteners. So, unlike other blankets, it can't fall off or become entangled in the stroller wheels. The stroller blanket is machine washable and not bulky, so it can be left on the stroller even when the stroller is folded up and put away.

- Cozy Rosie Stroller Blanket by Jeanette Benway
  Manufacturer Web site: *www.cozyrosie.com*
- Fleece Warmer by Kiddopotamus
  Vendor Web sites: *www.babies1st.com*; *www.babybungalow.com*
- Go Cozy by Kiddopotamus
  Vendor Web sites: *www.barebabies.com*; *www.babybungalow.com*

○ Stroller Connector

With stroller connectors, you can take two single umbrella strollers or two identical strollers and connect them together to make a double side-by-side stroller. This option is perfect for pushing two lightweight strollers at once. If you have two children but don't always want to take both of them with you at the same time, this device lets you have two single strollers instead of a larger double stroller. When you want to push both kids together, simply attach the two strollers with the connectors.

- Stroller Connectors by Prince Lionheart
  Manufacturer Web site: *www.princelionheart.com*

○ Stroller Extension Handle
For taller moms and dads who have ever had back pain or discomfort after a long day of stroller pushing, the stroller extension handle is the perfect invention. Personalize any stroller to your height with this adjustable attachment. Designed to offer one-handed stroller control, it allows busy parents on the go to multitask while keeping their children safe.

- Stroller Stretcher by Berkley Baby Products
  Manufacturer Web site: *www.strollerstretcher.com*
- SafeFit Stroller Handle Helpers
  Manufacturer Web site: *www.safefit.com*

Stroller Travel Bags

Everyday running around, not to mention traveling by plane or train, can take a toll on your stroller. Travel bags protect your stroller from damage and make it easy to transport standard, umbrella, and double strollers to any destination. The travel bag also keeps strollers free from dust and dirt when they're not in use.

○ Single-Stroller Travel Bags

- Carry Bag by Maclaren
  Manufacturer Web site: *www.maclarenbaby.com*
- Stroller Carrier for Standard/Dual Strollers by J. L. Childress
  Manufacturer Web site: *www.jlchildress.com*
- Stroller Cover'n Carry by Safefit
  Manufacturer Web site: *www.safefit.com*

○ Twin-Stroller Travel Bags

- Carry Bag by Maclaren
  Manufacturer Web site: *www.maclarenbaby.com*
- Stroller Carrier for Standard/Dual Strollers by J. L. Childress
  Manufacturer Web site: *www.jlchildress.com*
- Stroller Cover'n Carry by Safefit
  Manufacturer Web site: *www.safefit.com*

○ Umbrella-Stroller Travel Bags

- Padded Umbrella Stroller Travel Bag by J. L. Childress
  Manufacturer Web site: *www.jlchildress.com*
- Tote 'Ums by Leachco
  Manufacturer Web site: *www.leachco.com*

All fifty states require that parents have a car seat that meets federal safety standards before their baby may leave the hospital. It's the law for a reason. A correctly used car seat can reduce the chance of serious injury by 70 percent. All children are required to ride securely buckled in an infant car seat/carrier, convertible car seat, booster seat, or with a seat belt, whatever is appropriate for their weight and size. Before you buy a car seat, check the label to make sure the seat you choose meets current federal safety standards.

Once you have decided on a car seat for your child, read all the instructions for installation. Make sure they are clear and easy to understand to ensure proper installation in your car. If you are not sure how to install the car seat, take it to your local police or fire department, and someone there will properly install it for you.

When you buy a new car seat, be sure to send the registration card to the manufacturer so you will be notified of any problems or recalls.

FEATURES TO LOOK FOR

✔ Five-Point Harness

Safety experts recommend the five-point harness method of restraint as the safest. A five-point harness consists of a strap over each shoulder, one on each side of the pelvis, and one between the legs. All five straps come together at a common buckle. The harness should be made of wide, thick webbing and should lie flat against your child's body to distribute the force, in case of a crash, over a larger surface area. Narrow straps can become twisted and apply too much pressure in the wrong places, causing additional injury that could include cutting into your child's body.

✔ Easy-to-Adjust Harness Straps

Front-adjusting harness straps will make it easier to properly secure your baby in the car seat.

✔ Higher Weight Limit

Several convertible seats are now available with higher weight limits for bigger babies. Look for a seat that can be used by rear-facing babies up to 30 or 35 pounds.

✔ Reclining Seat

A reclining seat is much more comfortable for a newborn. A reclining seat also encourages napping. Look for easy-access levers or other adjustment devices.

✔ Canopy

The canopy will protect baby from the sun when he's riding in the back of the vehicle.

✔ Handle Adjustment

Many infant seats have adjustable ergonomic handles. Full-grip, padded handles and several locking positions are desirable for maximum comfort.

✔ Infant Head Support
An infant head support cradles your baby and provides added comfort and support.

✔ Energy-Absorbing Foam
A foam-covered car seat shell gives impact protection.

✔ Tether Strap
A tether is a strap that hooks the top of the car safety seat to a special permanent anchor in the vehicle called a tether anchor. Most anchors are located on the rear window ledge, the back of the vehicle seat, the floor, or the ceiling. Tethers give extra protection by keeping the car safety seat and the child's head from being thrown too far forward in a crash. The tether strap can be used in addition to the vehicle seat belt to reduce the chance of injury to your child. All new cars, minivans, and light trucks since September 2000 have been required to have upper tether anchors for securing the tops of car safety seats.

✔ Built-In Locking Clips
These clips eliminate the need to use separate locking clips. Locking clips are particularly helpful if your seat will be moved from car to car frequently.

✔ Seat Level Indicator
A level indicator ensures the car seat is installed at the proper angle.

✔ LATCH
LATCH (Lower Anchors and Tethers for Children) is a new car safety-seat attachment system that has been developed to make car safety seats easier to use. This new anchor system makes correct installation much easier because you will no longer need to use seat belts to secure the car safety seat. All cars, minivans, pickup trucks, and car safety seats made after September 2002 come with LATCH. However, unless both the vehicle and the car safety seat have this new anchor system, you will still need seat belts to secure the car safety seat.

✔ Easy-to-Clean Fabric
Children are messy, and car seats get dirty. Removable, machine-washable padding, pad covers, and canopies make life much easier.

✔ Separate Base and Removable Seat
This combination means you don't have to install the car seat every time you use it.

✔ Portability
Many car seats are approved for airline use, and some are even designed to rest securely in shopping carts.

○ Infant Car Seats/Carriers
If your child is less than one year old, no matter what his weight, he needs to ride in a rear-facing car seat. Newborns also should ride where adults can see them. Infant car seats/carriers are small, portable, and fit newborns

best. These units are designed for babies who weigh up to 20 to 22 pounds, depending on the model. They install rear facing in the back seat, the safest position for your baby. Even though starting off with a convertible-style car seat might seem more economical, an infant-only car seat will be safer for your baby. The crotch straps and harness straps will be closer to the baby's body to provide a better fit. The following car seats have all the features and safety recommendations previously listed.

- Companion Infant Car Seat by Britax
  Manufacturer Web site: *www.britaxusa.com*
  The Companion is a rear-facing infant carrier, with enhanced side-impact protection in the form of a head pad with adjustable, air-filled pockets that expand for a customized fit for each child.

- Embrace Premier Infant Car Seat by Evenflo
  Manufacturer Web site: *www.evenflo.com*
  This infant car seat is specially designed for Mom's comfort. The seat features an easy-carry, Z-shaped handle with soft overmold grip. The one-hand harness adjustment lets you properly position baby in the seat. Its Comfort Touch padding, three shoulder harness positions, and separate canopy make the Embrace Premier Infant Car Seat a luxurious choice for your baby.

- Primo Viaggio SIP Car Seat by Peg Perego
  Manufacturer Web site: *www.perego.com*
  This is a beautiful, top-quality car seat with a base that adjusts for the perfect fit. Just turn a dial on the base front to adjust the seat, and a side level tells you when you've got the right angle. Use this seat with any new model Peg Perego stroller, except the Aria twin.

- SnugRide Infant Car Seat by Graco
  Manufacturer Web site: *www.gracobaby.com*
  This car seat is top rated for safety and ease of use by leading consumer magazines. The car seat is outfitted with a cold-weather boot for extra warmth on chilly days. The five-point harness can be adjusted from the front of the seat to accommodate any type of baby clothing, for a proper fit every time.

○ Convertible Car Seats
Convertible car seats are bigger and heavier than infant-only car seats and are designed to grow with your child through the toddler years. These seats convert from five-point harness seats to belt-positioning booster seats. Convertible seats install rear or front facing, depending on the age and size of the child. A one-year-old child who sits unsupported and is taller than 26 inches and weighs at least 20 pounds can be moved into a forward-facing standard or convertible car seat. These seats are not designed to be taken in and out of the car, carried around, or snapped into a stroller.

- Alpha Omega Elite 5-Point Car Seat by Cosco
  Manufacturer Web site: *www.djgusa.com*
  The award-winning Alpha Omega is three car seats in one. It adapts from a rear-facing infant seat that accommodates babies up to 35 pounds to a front-facing toddler seat for children up to 40 pounds, and then to a child's booster seat for children up to 80 pounds. The included video and tether simplify installation.
- ComfortSport by Graco
  Manufacturer Web site: *www.gracobaby.com*
  The ComfortSport is the perfect transition car seat when your child has outgrown the infant car seat. This seat converts from rear-facing (5 pounds to 30 pounds) to forward-facing (20 pounds to 40 pounds). The removable snack/cup holders on both seat sides provide perfect storage for juice, crackers, and small toys.
- Roundabout by Britax
  Manufacturer Web site: *www.britaxusa.com*
  The legendary Britax Roundabout convertible car seat is renowned for safety, comfort, and convenience. The built-in LATCH system helps protect children by keeping seats more secure in vehicles. Roundabout accommodates babies in a rear-facing position from 5 pounds to 33 pounds, and older children in the forward-facing position up to 40 pounds. *Note:* The base of this seat is larger than most and may not fit in all cars properly.

The Roundabout is a fantastic car seat. It's easy to install and doesn't budge. I highly recommended it.—Betty

- Triumph 5 Convertible Car Seat by Evenflo
  Manufacturer Web site: *www.evenflo.com*
  This convertible car seat is taller and wider than most other convertible seats, to provide more room for your growing child. It has a compact base that actually fits better in most vehicles than many other convertible car seats on the market. As an added feature, the base of the car seat is designed to protect your car's upholstery. Triumph accommodates babies in a rear-facing position from 5 pounds to 30 pounds, and older children from 20 pounds to 40 pounds.
- Toddler/Booster Car Seats
  These seats are for children who are taller than 40 inches, weigh 30 pounds or more, and are not big enough to be safely restrained by adult seat belts alone.

Boosters have a high back and install front facing in the rear seat. Boosters must be used with both lap and shoulder belts.

- Parkway Booster Seat by Britax

  Manufacturer Web site: *www.britaxusa.com*

  Featuring wraparound side wings and a headrest area with EPS foam, the Parkway offers additional side-impact protection for your child in the event of a side-impact crash. The Parkway fits children who are from 38 inches to 60 inches tall and who weigh approximately 30 pounds to 100 pounds.

- High Back Booster Car Seat by Cosco

  Vendor Web site: *www.djgusa.com*

  This high-back booster provides extended use by accommodating children up to 100 pounds. Its three-position recline provides greater comfort for your child. The car seat features molded-in storage compartments with a slide-out cup holder. It includes a five-point internal harness for children 22 pounds to 40 pounds, and a belt-positioning booster for children 30 pounds to 100 pounds.

- TurboBooster SafeSeat by Graco

  Manufacturer Web site: *www.gracobaby.com*

  The sporty TurboBooster SafeSeat features a reversible knit/fleece pad for your child's comfort. The easy-to-adjust headrest features EPS energy-absorbing foam. Kids are sure to love the armrests, and the hideaway cup holders on either side of the seat are perfect for storing drinks, snacks, and toys. The TurboBooster is for children three years to ten years old, 30 pounds to 100 pounds in weight, and between 38 inches and 57 inches tall.

- Ultra CarGo Booster Car Seat by Graco

  Manufacturer Web site: *www.gracobaby.com*

  The deep, wide sides and high back of this car seat provide plenty of room, as well as back and head support, for your growing toddler. Your child will enjoy the convenient cup holder and mesh pocket for storing all kinds of kids' gear. For children 20 pounds to 40 pounds, the five-point harness fits securely across the hips. For children 30 pounds to 100 pounds, remove the harness, and the car seat becomes a belt-positioning booster.

Car Seat/Carrier Accessories

The following list contains products to protect baby from the elements, keep the car seat from getting too hot, provide support for baby's head and body, keep baby warm, organize necessities, protect the car seat from getting dirty, and more.

○ Infant Car Seat Covers
Protect baby from the elements with one of these infant car seat covers. The covers fit all standard infant carriers/car seats with a canopy.

- Baby Carrier Shield—Summer by Dex
  Vendor Web sites: *www.babyant.com; www.babybungalow.com*
  This cover protects baby from the sun, wind, and insects.

- Baby Carrier Shield—Winter by Dex
  Vendor Web sites: *www.babyant.com; www.babybungalow.com*
  This cover protects baby from severe cold, rain, wind, and insects.

- Infant Car Seat Netting by Graco
  Vendor Web sites: *www.babyage.com; www.babyuniverse.com*
  The netting protects baby from insects and mosquitoes.

○ Back-Seat Mirrors for Rear-Facing Car Seats
A back-seat mirror will give you peace of mind, letting you safely view your rear-facing baby while you're driving. Just by glancing in your rearview mirror, you will be able to see whatever your baby is doing.

- Baby In-Sight Mirror by SafeFit
  Manufacturer Web site: *www.safefit.com*
  This jumbo back seat mirror allows for greater visibility of your rear-facing infant. The mirror is great for any car, but it's a must-have for vans or large SUVs. The mirror is shatterproof for baby's safety.

- Baby Night Sight Mirror by SafeFit
  Manufacturer Web site: *www.safefit.com*
  Safely view your rear-facing infant day or night. Clip the remote control to your visor. Then look in the mirror, press the remote control, and the soft light gently illuminates baby's face for eight seconds before it automatically shuts off. The mirror is shatterproof for baby's safety.

- Deluxe Auto Mirror with Music & Lights by Fisher Price
  Manufacturer Web site: *www.fisher-price.com*
  This unique mirror allows Mom to safely and easily keep an eye on her rear-facing infant while it entertains baby with music and lights.

- Easy View Back Seat Mirror by Sunshine Kids
  Vendor Web sites: *www.kidsurplus.com; www.onestepahead.com*
  Unlike stationary baby car mirrors, this one is attached to a 360 rotating socket that lets you set the perfect angle to view your baby. In one glance you can see the road and baby too.

○ Car Mirrors for Front-Facing Car Seats
These mirrors securely attach to your car's rearview mirror, allowing you to view your baby at a glance.

- Baby-in-View Auto Mirror by Munchkin
  Manufacturer Web site: *www.munchkininc.com*

This mirror lets parents keep an eye on baby without adjusting the standard rear-view mirror. The mirror attaches to the front or back window with suctions cups, adjusts to any angle, and rotates 360 degrees to keep baby in sight.

- Baby on Board Flip-Down Child View Mirror by Safety 1st
Manufacturer Web site: *www.safety1st.com*
This accessory mirror attaches securely to your car's rearview mirror. It's easily adjustable so you can see your child at a glance.

- Baby on Board Front or Back Babyview Mirror by Safety 1st
Manufacturer Web site: *www.safety1st.com*
Use this mirror for rear-facing infants or clip it to the visor to view forward-facing children.

- 2-in-1 Wide Angle Mirror by SafeFit
Manufacturer Web site: *www.safefit.com*
This wide angle mirror provides a view of the entire back seat, which is great if you have multiple passengers. It can be used for rear-facing infants or forward-facing children.

○ Sunshades
Sunshades keep the sun out of baby's eyes, but not the view. Sunshades also help keep baby cooler and provide protection from the sun's harmful rays. The see-through material helps the driver see out of the window. Many sunshades can be raised or lowered by the simple push of a button.

- Baby on Board SunShade by Safety 1st
Manufacturer Web site: *www.safety1st.com*

- Rear Window Shade by Kel-Gar
Manufacturer Web site: *www.kelgar.com*

- Side Window Shade by Kel-Gar
Manufacturer Web site: *www.kelgar.com*

- Baby on Board Super Roller Shade by Safety 1st
Manufacturer Web site: *www.safety1st.com*

○ Head Supports
Pediatricians recommend greater support for tiny newborns and growing infants. Newborns and young babies can't hold their heads up by themselves until they are a few months old. Head supports protect your baby's head and neck. They keep your baby's head from falling to the side or flopping forward. Head supports provide extra support in car seats and carriers to keep baby stabilized and comfortable. You also can use head supports in infant seats, swings, and strollers. If you do not own a car seat with a built-in head support, here are some suggestions.

- Rainbow Wrap by Leachco
Manufacturer Web site: *www.leachco.com*

- Infant Head Support & Harness Covers Combo Pack by Graco
  Manufacturer Web site: *www.gracobaby.com*
- Double Headrest by Babies "R" Us
  Manufacturer Web site: *www.babiesrus.com*
- Prop-O's Head Support & Strap Cover by Leachco
  Manufacturer Web site: *www.leachco.com*

○ Total-Body Supports
Many child seats do not provide the total-body support an infant or toddler needs. A total-body support will cradle and support your baby's whole body for a more secure and comfortable ride. You can also use total-body supports in infant seats, swings, and strollers.

- Snuzzler by Kiddopotamus
  Manufacturer Web site: *www.kiddopotamus.com*
  Plush, cozy fleece provides the ultimate in year-round comfort with this support. Simply set the support into the seat. The Snuzzler fits every harness system, with no need to rethread shoulder straps.
- 3 Piece Total Body Support Set by Infantino
  Vendor Web sites: *www.babiesexpress.com*; *www.babyant.com*
  The 3 Piece Total Body Support Set lets you customize support for your baby. Baby's head, neck, and upper body are supported by side cushions. Reversible fabric keeps baby cool. The Total Body Support Set fits in the car seat, stroller, bouncer, jogger, or infant swing.

○ Car-Seat Strap Covers
Strap covers encircle the shoulder straps on baby's car seat or carrier to protect her tender skin from harsh chafing and rubbing.

- Cushy Straps Cushioned Strap Covers by Kiddopotamus
  Manufacturer Web site: *www.kiddopotamus.com*
- Deluxe Strap Covers by NoJo
  Vendor Web sites: *www.babycatalog.com*; *www.kidsurplus.com*

○ Car-Seat Canopy
Convertible and booster car seats don't come with one, but you can protect your baby from the hot sun with a canopy. This canopy easily attaches and removes with two clips. When your child is comfortable in the car, everyone will have a better ride.

- Combi Car Seat Canopy
  Vendor Web sites: *www.babyage.com*; *www.livingincomfort.com*

○ Car-Seat Bunting
Maintaining a constant body temperature is a necessity for babies. A sudden rise or drop in body temperature can adversely affect infants, especially preemies and newborns. You can keep baby comfortable in all types of weather, rain or shine, with a car-seat bunting. Car-seat buntings fit into car seats and eliminate

the need for blankets or bulky clothing. Buntings come in various fabrics, and some are reversible, so you can use the right side according to the season.

- CozyUp by Kiddopotamus
  Manufacturer Web site: *www.kiddopotamus.com*
- Original Bundle Me by J.J. Cole
  Vendor Web sites: *www.babiesrus.com*; *www.babyuniverse.com*

○ Car-Seat Organizers
Keep your car tidy with a back-seat organizer. Keep all of baby's necessities, toys, and games in one place.

- Backseat Organizer by Kel-Gar
  Manufacturer Web site: *www.kelgar.com*
  This easy-to-clean, multipocket storage system features a fold-down drink holder and tray and fits over any vehicle seat headrest.
- Sort & Go Portable Organizer by Infantino
  Manufacturer Web site: *www.infantino.com*
  This organizer's large storage pockets hold all of baby's favorite things.
- Stuff N Scuff by The Right Start
  Manufacturer Web site: *www.therightstart.com*
  Protect your seat from little feet. The Stuff N Scuff fastens easily around any headrest, and the large cargo pocket holds everything.

○ Car-Seat Protector
A car-seat protector keeps baby's car seat neat and easy to clean.

- Piddle Pad Waterproof Seat Liner by Kiddopotamus
  Manufacturer Web site: *www.kiddopotamus.com*
  The Piddle Pad is made of soft, absorbent seat fabric for baby's comfort. Contoured, yet foldable and flexible, the Piddle Pad easily and discreetly fits into every child's seat, from newborns to toddlers.

○ Car-Seat Shields
Sitting outside, unprotected from the sun, baby's car seat can get very hot. Touching hot car-seat parts can cause serious burns to baby's skin. Keep your car seat cooler and your child safer by using a car-seat shield. Sun shields fold easily and fit into their own compact pocket.

- Car Seat Shade by Prince Lionheart
  Manufacturer Web site: *www.princelionheart.com*

I purchased this car seat shade by Prince Lionheart for a trip to Arizona and it worked out beautifully. My daughter's car seat stayed cool and I didn't have to worry about hot buckles. —Pam

- Sun Stop'r Car Seat Cover by Kel-Gar
  Manufacturer Web site: *www.kelgar.com*

○ Car-Seat Mobile
Captivate and entertain baby on the go. This suction-cup mobile adheres to the side window and moves with the motion of the car.

- ZooMobile by Infantino
  Manufacturer Web site: *www.infantino.com*

○ Vehicle Upholstery Protectors for a Single Car Seat
Babies can be messy. Protect your vehicle's upholstery from scuffs and spills with a waterproof upholstery protector. Upholstery protectors prevent difficult cleanups and frustrating stains from occurring.

- Auto Seat Protector by Munchkin
  Manufacturer Web site: *www.munchkininc.com*
  A specially designed stabilizing wedge keeps the Auto Seat Protector securely in place and contours it to fit any car seat. The handy front storage pocket keeps baby's essentials neat and nearby.

- Especially for Baby Car Seat Undermat by Sassy
  Vendor Web site: *www.babiesrus.com*
  The Car Seat Undermat works with all infant/child car seats and is LATCH compatible. Three mesh storage pockets drape down over the seat to keep toys and supplies organized.

- Grip & Go Non-Slip Seat Protector by Infantino
  Manufacturer Web site: *www.princelionheart.com*
  This non-slip seat cover slides under forward- or rear-facing car seats and protects upholstery from scuffs, spills, and compression marks. Three roomy pockets are perfect for storing everything baby needs for a short or long trip.

- Two-Stage Seatsaver by Prince Lionheart
  Manufacturer Web site: *www.princelionheart.com*
  Use the bottom tray alone with rear-facing infant car seats. The back attaches to the bottom tray for use with forward-facing toddler and booster car seats. This seatsaver's high-density foam construction prevents depression damage to your vehicle's seats.

○ Car-Seat Travel Bags
Baby's car seat is always difficult to carry when you're traveling. A car-seat travel bag will protect your car seat from dirt and damage, and it is the most convenient way to transport the car seat to your travel destination. If you are traveling by plane, you can check the car seat as luggage and not have to worry about it. Zippered storage bags have convenient handles and shoulder straps for comfortable carrying, and the travel bags wipe clean with a damp sponge.

- 2-in-1 Car Seat Cover'n Carry by SafeFit (car-seat travel tote and sunshade)
  Manufacturer Web site: *www.safefit.com*
- Ultimate Car Seat/Booster Seat Carrier by J. L. Childress
  Manufacturer Web site: *www.jlchildress.com*
- Wheelie Car Seat Travel Bag by J. L. Childress
  Manufacturer Web site: *www.jlchildress.com*

SLINGS, CARRIERS, AND BACKPACKS

Sometimes a stroller is not the best way to travel. Babies don't always need wheels to get around in style. A sling, carrier, or backpack gives your baby a different perspective than a stroller, and it keeps him close, which fosters a parent-child bond. One advantage of using a sling, carrier, or backpack is that it leaves your hands free and keeps your child close to you. These options make navigating stairs, crowded stores, busy sidewalks, subway stations, and buses easier. But before you buy any type of carrier, try it on to make sure it's comfortable for both you and your baby.

○ Slings

Slings are best for carrying newborns under 20 pounds. Slings are simply a wide piece of fabric that hangs across an adult's torso and is supported by a shoulder strap. Slings satisfy both the physical and emotional needs of mother and baby. Slings let baby rest in a comfortable, natural sleeping position. They hold baby close and allow for flexible nursing positions. Slings are great for carrying a fussy newborn around the house or taking her for a short walk.

- Maya Wrap by Maya Wrap
  Manufacturer Web site: *www.mayawrap.com*
- 100% Regular Cotton Baby Carrier by New Native
  Manufacturer Web site: *www.newnativebaby.com*
- Over the Shoulder Baby Holder
  Manufacturer Web site: *www.babyholder.com*

○ Front/Back Carriers

Carriers are made up of two shoulder straps that support a fabric seat. They have adjustable settings to help distribute your baby's weight across your back and shoulders. Most carriers hold newborns facing your chest. When your baby has sufficient head control, you can turn him to face forward so he can get a good view. Some carriers switch from front to back so you can carry a small baby against your chest, and then use the carrier as a backpack when your child is six months old and older. Snuggled next to you in a front carrier, baby will stay warm. Pick a carrier made of cotton or other breathable fabric that won't make baby too hot. Also, make sure the carrier has a sturdy headrest to support a sleeping baby's head and neck. Seat and leg holes should be banded with a soft fabric that won't irritate baby's delicate skin. Leg holes should adjust to accommodate a newborn and lock into a safe, fixed position. A side-entry access on the carrier will make it easier to get baby in and out.

- Baby Björn Active Carrier by Baby Björn
  Vendor Web sites: *www.babiesrus.com*; *www.babycenter.com*; *www.target.com*
  This carrier is easy to put on and take off because all adjustments are made in front. The carrier grows with baby, thanks to an adjustable buckle that gives comfort for all ages. Its design even lets you breast-feed without removing the baby. If baby falls asleep in the Björn, simply unsnap the front piece and lay baby down without waking him up!

- Kangaroo Carrier by Kelty
  Manufacturer Web site: *www.kelty.com*
  This carrier features a zip-off storage sack for bottles and diapers. The zip-out hood protects baby from the elements and provides privacy for nursing. The carrier accommodates babies from three weeks to twelve months old.

- Maclaren Techno Baby Carrier
  Manufacturer Web site: *www.maclarenbaby.com*
  The Maclaren Techno carrier outshines other carriers because of its unique, removable "pod" to cradle babies weighing 8 pounds to 12 pounds. A secondary restraint belt ensures that baby is safely in place. This carrier is uniquely designed so baby can be safely inserted on a flat surface, such as a parent's lap.

○ Infant Carrier for Multiples

- MaxiMom—Multiple Births Baby Carrier by Tot Tenders
  Vendor Web sites: *www.babiesexpress.com*; *www.4coolkids.com*
  The MaxiMom is a unique carrier that works in nine different positions. The variety of positions and the ease of use make this a great carrier for twins and even triplets. Babies can be forward facing or chest facing. They can be carried on the back or the side. You can place the babies side by side, or one in the front and one in the back. Each baby can be attached or detached to and from you individually, which allows for more flexibility. The carrier stays with the baby in the car seat or on the shopping cart, or it can be used as an emergency highchair.

○ Backpack Carriers
When your child outgrows his carrier, you might want to consider a backpack, especially if you are trekking on unfriendly stroller terrain. Your baby should be able to sit up alone, though, before she rides in a backpack. A baby backpack has a seat for baby, supported by a lightweight frame. Backpacks are best worn for longer excursions. If you are making a lot of stops and need to take the backpack off at each destination, it can become tedious. When you're buying a backpack, look for one with a waist belt to take the pressure off your back and

shoulders. A backpack with a frame that stands on its own will be easier to pull on and off when you are alone. The backpack should be lightweight, and have an adjustable inside seat and a harness that will safely strap baby in—preferably one that fits across baby's chest and shoulders. If you plan to use your backpack year-round, look for brands that have optional add-ons such as sun canopies. A model that has pockets provides a convenient place for necessities.

- Adventure by Kelty
  Manufacturer Web site: *www.kelty.com*
  For parents who consider backpacking and hiking an essential experience, Kelty's top-of-the-line Adventure carrier makes it easy to introduce your baby to the outdoors. Features include a five-point harness, climbing-rope handles, toy loops, removable kid pack with shoulder straps, a sun/rain hood, and an auto-deploy kickstand. The carrier weighs 8 pounds 4 ounces and accommodates a child who weighs up to 40 pounds.

- Pathfinder Frame Carrier by Kelty
  Manufacturer Web site: *www.kelty.com*
  This carrier is great for strolling around town or hiking. Features include a five-point harness, padded shoulder straps, a sun/rain hood to keep your baby comfortable in any kind of weather, toy loops, a removable kid pack, and an auto-deploy kickstand. The carrier weighs 7.75 pounds and accommodates a child up to 50 pounds.

- Tour Frame Carrier by Kelty
  Manufacturer Web site: *www.kelty.com*
  The Tour Frame Carrier is a sturdy, easy-to-use, lightweight backpack that's ideal for everyday use. Features include a five-point harness, a height-adjustable seat, adjustable padded parents straps, a large storage pocket for baby's supplies, and toy loops for keeping pacifiers and small toys within easy reach. This carrier weighs 4.75 pounds and accommodates a child up to 50 pounds.

○ Stroller Backpacks
Stroller backpacks are the perfect solution for parents on the go: the convenience of a child carrier and stroller in one product. The units convert from a backpack to a stroller in seconds.

- Convertible Stroller Pack by Kelty
  Vendor Web sites: *www.babyage.com*; *www.babyuniverse.com*
  The Convertible Stroller Pack is perfect for travel, the mall, amusement parks, or any situation in which mobility and convenience are a priority. When the convertible is used as a carrier, the wheel cover protects the parents from dirty wheels. Other features include a five-point harness; a two-layer, one-piece curved waist belt; a mesh back panel; and padded shoulder straps. The stroller weighs 9 pounds 3 ounces and accommodates a child up to 45 pounds.

Chapter 23

Traveling Accessories

When you're out and about, it's important to have everything you need for baby's comfort. Baby might get hungry or need a diaper change or a place to sleep. You will want to keep baby's bottle and food cold until he's ready to eat, and then be able to warm them up at feeding time. You'll want a clean, sanitary place to change your baby, and a nice, safe place for him to sleep. When you're traveling around, these products will afford you all the comforts of home.

FEEDING ON THE GO

Baby can get hungry anytime or anywhere. When that happens, you want to be ready, and you want to be sure cold foods stay cold and warm foods stay warm until baby's ready to eat.

○ Insulated Bottle and Food Bags
When you are away from home, you want to make sure baby's bottles and food stay at just the right temperature so they won't spoil. Insulated bottles and food bags come in various sizes and with reusable ice packs to keep bottles and food cold until baby's ready to eat.

  ● Avent Thermal Tote by Avent
    Manufacturer Web site: *www.aventamerica.com*
    This stylish tote holds Avent bottles, VIA Disposables, or Magic Cups and maintains the correct temperature for on-the-go feeding. The Thermal Tote has a handy front pocket for snacks and a zippered main compartment easily holds bottles or cups.

  ● Cup 'n Stuff Stroller Pocket by J. L. Childress
    Manufacturer Web site: *www.jlchildress.com*
    This handy travel bag attaches to any stroller and provides space for cups, bottles, snacks, and your cell phone. The bag

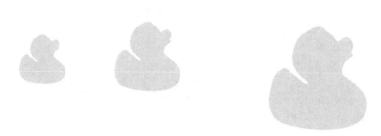

attaches to the stroller handle or bumper bar for easy child access. The nonslip strap prevents the bag from slipping or wiggling when the stroller moves over bumpy ground.

- Mealtime Tote by The First Years
  Manufacturer Web site: *www.thefirstyears.com*
  The Mealtime Tote holds three 8-ounce bottles and three 4-ounce jars at just the right temperature. The snap handles fit strollers.

- Multi-Purpose MaxiCool by J. L. Childress
  Manufacturer Web site: *www.jlchildress.com*
  This cooler holds four standard-size bottles or three Avent bottles. The MaxiCool includes front and back pockets for small items, and a new ID card and pocket. The snap handle attaches to all strollers.

- "6 Bottle Cooler" by J. L. Childress
  Manufacturer Web site: *www.jlchildress.com*
  This cooler is perfect for a full day's supply of baby's feeding needs, and it's great if you have multiples. The unit holds six standard bottles, or three bottles and a cereal box. The top compartment holds three food jars, utensils, and bibs. The cooler features a back pocket and an ID card and pocket.

○ Extra Hot and Cool Gel Packs
  Keep extra hot and cool gel packs in the freezer, ready to keep baby's food cool and fresh for hours, or warm and ready to use. You can microwave extra gel packs and place them with diaper wipes to keep them warm for those diaper changes away from home.

  - Hot & Cold Gel Pak by Prince Lionheart
    Manufacturer Web site: *www.princelionheart.com*

- Hot & Cool Gel Packs by J. L. Childress
  Manufacturer Web site: *www.jlchildress.com*

○ Bottle Holder
  Keep your baby's bottle close at hand with a bottle holder. And with a bottle holder, you'll have no more of dropping baby's bottle on the ground or losing it between the seats in the car.

  - Bottle Keeper by Mommy's Helper
    Vendor Web sites: *www.babyant.com*; *www.babybungalow.com*
    This holder's hook and loop fastener lets you attach the Bottle Keeper to a highchair, stroller, car seat, or other convenient location. The holder fits regular bottles, angled bottles, and most nonspill sippy cups.

○ Disposable Placemats
  Disposable placemats provide your child with a clean, sanitary eating surface wherever you go.

  - Table Toppers Placemats by Neat Solutions
    Manufacturer Web site: *www.neatsolutions.com*
    Each disposable placemat adheres to a table surface with adhesive strips to ensure that your child eats on a sanitary surface.

  - TravelWare Disposable Placemats by Munchkin
    Manufacturer Web site: *www.munchkininc.com*
    These handy disposable placemats have nonslip adhesive strips so they always stay put, and the superabsorbent quilted fabric is backed with a special leakproof liner, so no matter what baby eats, the table stays neat.

Portable Bottle Warmers

Baby can have warm milk and food anywhere you go, just like at home. There are two types of portable bottle warmers: the automobile bottle warmer, and the wraparound bottle warmer.

○ Vehicle Adapter Bottle Warmers
  Plug the bottle warmer into your car adapter outlet, and your baby has a warm bottle in minutes. These warmers fit all baby bottles and food jars. The bottle warmers have on/off switches for added safety. The warmers fit in cup holders. Warmers are not recommended for disposable bottles.

  - Automobile Bottle Warmer by Dex
    Manufacturer Web site: *www.dexproducts.com*

  - Car Bottle Warmer By Munchkin
    Manufacturer Web site: *www.munchkininc.com*

○ Wraparound Bottle Warmers
  Now, with a touch of a button, you can heat a bottle or baby food jar no matter where you go. No batteries or electrical supply are needed. Just wrap the

heat pack of the bottle warmer around your bottle or baby food jar, insert the unit into the insulated bag, and the heating process will begin.

- Heater Wrap Portable Bottle Warmer by J. L. Childress
  Vendor Web sites: *www.baby-hugs.com*; *www.babyproofingplus.com*; *www.greatbeginningsonline.com*
- On-the-Go Bottle Warmer by Prince Lionheart
  Manufacturer Web site: *www.princelionheart.com*

○ Portable Food Bowl
Now you don't have to feed baby out of a jar. A portable food bowl not only gives you a clean place to put baby's food, but also lets you dish out just the right amount of food for each feeding.

- Folding Bowl by Gerber Children's Products
  Manufacturer Web site: *www.gerber.com*
  The Folding Bowl is a two-compartment bowl that holds food or two baby food jars on one side, and eating utensils and bib on the other side. The bowl folds in half for easy storage.

I think the Gerber Folding Bowl is a great product. You have everything right there: the bowl, food, spoon and a bib. I love how compact it is as well.—Olivia

DIAPER CHANGING

Changing baby's diaper becomes a familiar routine at home. But when you're out and about and it's time for a change, the process can be more challenging without the proper accessories. Choose what you'll need from the following list to simplify diaper changing when you're away from home.

○ Diaper Holder
Keep diapers and wipes handy and organized for travel.

- Diapees & Wipees
  Manufacturer Web site: *www.diapeesandwipees.com*
  Say goodbye to wadded, scrunched-up diapers. Diapees & Wipees will keep your baby's diapers nice and neat, just like they came out of the package. Diapees & Wipees is designed specifically to hold a travel pack of wipes and two to four diapers. Use Diapees & Wipees with your diaper bag. Or when you want to lighten your load, just grab the Diapees & Wipees bag and go.

○ Portable Changing Pads
It's not always easy to find a clean, sanitary place to change your baby. A portable changing pad will solve that problem.

- Changing Pad Wallet by J. L. Childress
  Manufacturer Web site: *www.jlchildress.com*
  The Changing Pad Wallet is a full-size changing pad that folds to the size of a woman's wallet. Compact styling makes it the perfect accessory to all diaper bags.
- Full Body Changing Pad by J. L. Childress
  Manufacturer Web site: *www.jlchildress.com*
  Protect baby's entire body with this oversized changing pad. When it's folded, the changing pad conveniently fits in a purse, diaper bag, or travel bag. You can use the webbing strap to attach diapers or the wipe container to the changing pad.

SANITATION

Use the following products to help ensure baby's health when she's riding in the shopping cart.

○ Cloth Shopping-Cart Covers
  Babies love to teethe on shopping-cart handles. Shopping-cart covers will protect your child from the dangerous germs that lurk on unsanitary, unwashed shopping carts.

- Clean Shopper by Babe Ease
  Manufacturer Web site: *www.babeease.com*
  The Clean Shopper is designed to fit all standard grocery carts. The unique, one-piece design covers all metal and plastic surfaces of grocery-cart areas, so babies and toddlers are not exposed to metal and cannot touch or suck the cart's germ-ridden handlebars. The cover installs in seconds with one easy step. It includes a self-contained safety strap and buckle to help babies and toddlers sit securely in the seat.

My baby likes to chew on shopping-cart handles. I love the Clean Shopper. It covers the cart and I don't have to worry about him picking up germs.—Cindy

- Safe Shopper Set by Leachco
  Manufacturer Web site: *www.leachco.com*
  The Safe Shopper Set combines the Prop 'N Soft and Easy Teether Cart Handle for the ultimate in shopping safety. Both pieces are fully padded and adjustable with Velcro. The Prop 'N Soft provides the extra support baby needs for unexpected stops and turns and the handle cover includes two attachments for baby's special toys.

- Shop 'n' Dine by Baby Buddy
  Manufacturer Web site: *www.babybuddy.com*
  Shop 'n' Dine offers your child protection from unsanitary shopping cart handles and also provides a comfortable padded seat with a secure five-point harness system. You can use Shop 'n' Dine to create a secure and comfortable seat in those wooden highchairs you commonly find in restaurants.
- Disposable Shopping-Cart Handle Covers
  Disposable shopping-cart handle covers fit conveniently in your purse or diaper bag. Use them once and throw them away.
  - Shopper Topper by Neat Solutions
    Vendor Web sites: *www.babyage.com*; *www.kidsurplus.com*
    This sanitary and disposable shopping-cart handle cover protects children from germs on shopping cart handles. The cover sticks in place with adhesive strips. The cover's Activity Center educates and occupies your child while you shop.

SLEEPING

If you are going visiting, you need a safe place to put baby down for a nap. If you don't want to carry around a Pack 'N Play, here are some simple alternatives for newborns and infants. When baby can sit upright unaided, discontinue use of these products.

- Portable Travel Beds
  - Baby Travel Bed by Samsonite
    Vendor Web sites: *www.babybungalow.com*; *www.minitots.com*
    This portable bed includes a zippered, fitted terry sheet; mosquito netting cover that snaps to the bed; two zippered compartments, one insulated for bottles or food storage; and a mattress pad. The ergonomically adjustable shoulder carrying straps make the bed easy to take anywhere.
  - Nap N Pack by Leachco
    Manufacturer Web site: *www.leachco.com*
    The Nap N Pack opens up into a large napper that assembles in seconds. Easily attach all four Velcro side tabs, and the unit transforms to a full-size napper for newborns and infants.
  - 3 in 1 Genie by Dex
    Manufacturer Web site: *www.dexproducts.com*
    This is a product for parents on the go; it's a diaper bag, changing table, and a bed you can take anywhere. The Genie has a padded shoulder strap for comfort, and extra-large pockets store all of baby's essentials. The unit even includes insulated bottle and food sleeves.

Chapter 24
Toys for Baby's First Year

Toys play an important part in baby's development. They help build hand-eye coordination, stimulate senses, develop fine motor skills, and promote creativity.

TOY SAFETY TIPS
Before you buy any toy, here are a few safety tips to look for:

- ✔ Read the toy information before you purchase any toy. Make sure the toy is age appropriate for your baby.
- ✔ Check the toys for small pieces that young children can remove and swallow.
- ✔ Use a small-object tester to ensure that the pieces are not a choking hazard (see Chapter 8 for small-object testers).
- ✔ For young children, avoid toys with strings or ropes, which could be a strangulation hazard.
- ✔ Clean toys regularly, especially toys that come in contact with a child's mouth.
- ✔ Be careful with antique and old toys. The toys could have sharp edges and small pieces, or they might contain lead paint.
- ✔ If the toy has chipped paint or broken pieces, discard it.
- ✔ If the toy uses batteries, make sure the batteries are not easily accessible to children.
- ✔ If you have children of a different age group in the same household, separate the toys so that children cannot reach toys that are unsafe for their age group.
- ✔ Designate a play area where toys are kept to avoid accidents.
- ✔ All toys should be well constructed so they won't break apart.
- ✔ Follow all instructions on package and labels.

BLACK, WHITE, AND RED TOYS

When a baby is born, she can see your face when it's about six inches away, but she can't yet make out the features. During the first six weeks after birth, your baby's vision will mature, and she will have an innate attraction to bold, high-contrast colors and patterns. The first colors your baby will recognize are black, white, and red. High-contrast toys and playmats are designed to help your little one pick out the differences in shapes and patterns to stimulate her visual development. Black, white, and red toys are highly tempting for infants to gaze upon and reach for, which helps to develop their motor skills, as well. There are a variety of black, white, and red toys to keep baby stimulated and entertained while she's in the crib or car seat, or on the floor.

○ Black, White, and Red Toys

- Car Seat Gallery by Manhattan
  Attach the Car Seat Gallery to the back of your vehicle's front seat, and arrange the graphic cards in the four see-through pockets. As you drive, your baby can look at the back of your seat and study the cards to develop her thinking skills.
  Manufacturer Web site: *www.manhattanbaby.com*

- Double Sided First Book by Tiny Love
  This is a dual-stage developmental book. One side, for babies from birth to three months, has high-contrast black, white, and red illustrations to encourage visual stimulation. The other side, for babies from three months to six months, has brightly colored, more complex, raised 3D figures and activities.
  Manufacturer Web site: *www.tinylove.com*

- First Mirror by Lamaze
  Baby delights in learning to recognize her face in this mirror. The mirror has bright colors and flexible adapter straps that attach to crib or stroller.
  Manufacturer Web site: *www.learningcurve.com*
- Gymini 3D Activity Gym in Black, White, & Red by Tiny Love
  The Gymini's stimulating shapes, vivid colors, rattles, and musical melodies all keep baby occupied and happy with fun activities.
  Manufacturer Web site: *www.tinylove.com*
- Octopus Rattle—Black, White and Red by Tiny Love
  The Octopus Rattle has springy legs for baby to pull. You can add the rattle to the Gymini, Activity Arch, Take-Along Arch, and more.
  Manufacturer Web site: *www.tinylove.com*

CRIB TOYS

During the first year, babies spend a lot of time in their cribs. Crib toys help develop hand-eye coordination, are developmentally stimulating, and are a great source of entertainment. Some crib toys, such as Slumbertime Soothers, feature music, white noise, or sounds actually recorded in the womb to help send your little one off to dreamland.

- Plush Slumbertime Soothers
  - Mommy Bear by Dex
    Mommy Bear calms and comforts your baby to sleep with sounds recorded in the womb. Mommy Bear has an adjustable volume control and battery saver with an autoshutoff feature after forty minutes.
    Manufacturer Web site: *www.dexproducts.com*
  - Sleep Sheep by Cloudb
    Sleep Sheep features four soothing sounds—mother's heart-beat, spring showers, ocean surf, and whale songs. Sleep Sheep has a removable sound box with adjustable volume and on/off controls.
    Manufacturer Web site: *www.cloudb.com*
  - The Original Slumber Bear by Prince Lionheart
    Slumber Bear will lull your baby to sleep in minutes with sounds from the womb. Motion sensors reactivate the recording when baby moves.
    Manufacturer Web site: *www.princelionheart.com*

We bought the Slumber Bear for my son when he was having a hard time sleeping at night. It has worked wonders and now the bear is his best friend.—Sally

○ Musical Slumbertime Soothers

- Flutterbye Dreams Lullabye Birdies Soother by Fisher Price
  The birdies' fluttering motion is unique, and baby will be mesmerized.
  Add soothing music and nature sounds, soft light, and a ceiling light
  show of soothing nature scenes, and baby will drift off to Flutterbye
  Dreams.
  Manufacturer Web site: *www.fisher-price.com*

- Ocean Wonders Aquarium by Fisher Price
  Soothe baby to sleep with the sights and sounds of a mesmerizing
  aquarium. Swimming fish, gentle bubbles, and softly glowing lights join
  with calming music and serene aquatic sounds to lull baby to sleep.
  Manufacturer Web site: *www.fisher-price.com*

○ Musical Crib Toys

- Developlay Activity Center by Tiny Love
  The Developlay Activity Center will keep baby busy happily pulling,
  pushing, spinning, and grasping at the many activities on the play center. Age-appropriate activities, designed for different aspects of baby
  development, will help your baby, and soon, growing toddler, discover
  new challenges from about age three months to twenty-four months,
  making this a true grow-with-baby toy.
  Manufacturer Web site: *www.tinylove.com*

- Link-a-Doos Kick & Play Piano by Fisher Price
  When tiny feet touch the piano keys, it comes alive with sound and color.
  Tie the piano to the side of the crib. Newborns will be delighted with
  the continuous play of animal music and twinkling lights. Toddlers can sit
  and play with the piano on the floor, creating their own concerts.
  Manufacturer Web site: *www.fisher-price.com*

○ Soft Crib Toys

- Carousel Tiger Spiral by Manhattan Baby
  The Carousel Tiger Spiral features three dangling soft toys.
  Manufacturer Web site: *www.manhattanbaby.com*

- Pull 'n' Play Activity Arch by Tiny Love
  From birth to five months, the arch is used spanning the crib; then,
  from five months onward, it attaches to the side of the crib.
  Manufacturer Web site: *www.tinylove.com*

- Starz Lights & Sounds by Manhattan Baby
  Starz Lights & Sounds captivates children with multisensory activities.
  This brightly colored toy attaches to almost anything, from crib to
  stroller to car-seat handle. Combining visual and auditory stimuli, this
  toy features lights and plays "Twinkle, Twinkle, Little Star."
  Manufacturer Web site: *www.manhattanbaby.com*

CRIB MIRRORS

Create a stimulating interactive environment in your child's crib with a mirror. Babies love seeing their own faces. They will coo and smile at themselves with delight. A mirror will help develop your baby's visual discrimination and recognition skills. Crib mirrors attach to the side of your child's crib with adjustable straps, Velcro, or ribbons. Once your baby reaches the age of five months, or is able to pull up to a standing position, remove the mirror from the crib to prevent baby from using it as a step to climb out. Baby can then play with the mirror on the floor. Many crib mirrors are encased in a fabric wedge. Remove the mirror and use the wedge on the floor for tummy-time play.

○ Musical Crib Mirrors
- Music and Me Spinning Mirror by Lamaze
  The Music and Me Spinning Mirror will have baby giggling with delight. Flower petals have bright designs with mirrors, and little insect pals encourage baby to reach and touch, developing motor skills.
  Vendor Web sites: *www.albeebaby.com*; *www.teachingplanet.com*; *www.trains4tots.com*
- Ocean Wonders Musical Activity Mirror by Fisher Price
  Here's a large, shiny mirror to play peek-a-boo with, and three ocean characters for baby to play with.
  Manufacturer Web site: *www.fisher-price.com*
- Miracles & Milestones Rhymes-Go-Round Mirror by Fisher Price
  Attach this elephant-friend mirror to baby's crib, or move it to the floor for tummy-time or sit-up play.
  Manufacturer Web site: *www.fisher-price.com*

○ Non-Musical Crib Mirrors
- First Mirror by Lamaze
  With bright-colored fabric, this high-quality, unbreakable, baby-safe mirror has a soft wedge to support baby during tummy time.
  Manufacturer Web site: *www.learningcurve.com*
- Me in the Mirror by Sassy
  Colorful ribbons, rings, and toys invite gazing and touching with this mirror. The mirror angles down or hangs flat in crib for baby to see when she's lying down or sitting. For floor play, the mirror stands with its easel feature.
  Manufacturer Web site: *www.sassybaby.com*

MUSICAL PULL-STRING TOYS

Soft musical pull-string toys attach easily with plush ties, Velcro, or ribbon to crib rails, car seats, playpens, and strollers. Musical pull-string toys soothe and entertain your baby. Music and movement encourage sight and hearing development. Newborns will enjoy gazing at this musical toy and listening to a variety of lullabies and nursery rhymes. Toddlers will enjoy being able to make the toy work all by themselves.

- ○ Musical Pull-String Toys
  - • Carouse Bird Pull Musical by Manhattan Baby
    "Brahm's Lullaby" is activated when baby pulls on the bird's tail feathers.
    Manufacturer Web site: *www.manhattanbaby.com*
  - • Flatso Musical Pull Downs by North American Bear
    Flatso favorites not only adorn the crib but also peek over the edge and play soothing lullabies. Simply pull the pastel stuffed toy at the end of the cord, and it's off to dreamland.
    Vendor Web site: *www.babyant.com*
  - • Little Lovelies Musical by Manhattan Baby
    Little Lovelies Musical features a cute little piggy, an adorable bunny rabbit, and a soft little lamb. Beethoven's "Für Elise" plays when the bunny rabbit's string is pulled, to help develop baby's cause-and-effect understanding.
    Manufacturer Web site: *www.manhattanbaby.com*
  - • Whoozit Pull Musical by Manhattan Toy
    This colorful music maker plays "Twinkle, Twinkle, Little Star." A baby-safe mirror reflects light and motion, dangling objects encourage exploration, and bright graphics hold children's attention.
    Vendor Web sites: *www.babyant.com*; *www.toyscamp.com*

BATHTUB TOYS

Most babies love to take a bath. Playing in the water is one of their favorite things to do. And a bath is even more fun when there are toys to play with. Before you give your baby any bath toys, check them to make sure there are no loose pieces, small parts that your baby could put in his mouth, sharp edges that could cause scratches or cuts, holes that can catch little fingers, or pieces that can break off. Avoid large inflatable toys in the tub—they can trap a small toddler or child under water. And stay away from wooden toys; wood holds moisture that allows bacteria to grow. Here are a few bath toys that will make your baby giggle and laugh while he's taking a bath.

- ○ Bathtub Toys
  - • Aquatic Bobbers by Sassy
    Tap on the bobbers to see the fish and frog characters bobble back and forth. Show baby how to immerse the bobbers in water for silly sounds and a variety of water-straining activities.
    Manufacturer Web site: *www.sassybaby.com*

My six-month-old loves to play with these Aquatic Bobbers in the bath. They are fun and he loves to chew on them.—Hannah

- Chewy Ark by Infantino
  Your baby will love playing with the four colorful, squeaky animals and the ark. When bath time is over, all the pieces fit together like a puzzle.
  Vendor Web sites: *www.amazon.com; www.littlenoahsark.com*

- Counting Fish 'N Net by Sassy
  Baby can scoop and strain water with each little fish (and the net) while learning to count. Easy-to-grasp fish and fishing net are sized just for little hands. Each of the colored fish has a number and corresponding holes in the bottom to make scooping and straining water easy for baby.
  Manufacturer Web site: *www.sassybaby.com*

- Sea Squirts by Munchkin
  These five colorful, smiling, big-eyed sea creatures float happily in the tub until your child calls them into action. Squeeze them to fill with water, then squeeze again and watch them squirt.
  Manufacturer Web site: *www.munchkininc.com*

- Color Change Ducky by Safety 1st
  What would a bath be without a rubber ducky? This little ducky is perfect for the tub. If the water is too hot the color change seal reveals the word "HOT." It floats upright and is watertight, so moisture cannot build up inside.
  Manufacturer Web site: *www.safety1st.com*

- Squirting Sea Pals by Sassy
  Here's a trio of squirters! Squeeze the lobster and water squirts to spin the ball in its claws. The snail and starfish squirt water, too.
  Manufacturer Web site: *www.sassybaby.com*

- Water Symphony by Tomy
  Each of this set of eight dolphins plays a different note when tapped on the head, which leads to creative compositions in the bath. The dolphins can be hooked together by their inner tubes, or they can float freely.
  Vendor Web sites: *www.kidsurplus.com; www.onestepahead.com*

INFANT CAR SEAT/CARRIER TOYS

Babies spend a lot of time in their infant car seat/carriers. Without something to look at and play with, they can get pretty bored. These toys can provide entertainment for your baby while he's in the car, out for a walk in the stroller, or just sitting in the infant car seat/carrier at home. If you're going to visit family or friends, these are the perfect take-along toys. You'll have no extra pieces to carry because they're already attached to the infant car seat/carrier. If baby gets tired of sitting in the carrier, detach the toys from the toy bar and he can play with them separately. These toys also can be used on cribs and strollers.

○ Infant Car Seat/Carrier Toys

- Baby Neptune Carrier Toy Bar by Baby Einstein
The Baby Neptune Carrier Toy Bar features a brightly colored, water-filled wave tank that includes a bobbing starfish, turtle, and dolphin swimming to the melodies of Handel and Strauss. A baby-safe bead chaser provides added entertainment for your baby.
Manufacturer Web site: *www.babyeinstein.com*

- Link Along Friends by Lamaze
Three cute friends with links are easy to take with you when you're on the go. Pull the bug, and he wiggles and shakes. The turtle has teether tabs to chew on. The octopus makes fun squeaky noises and has an eye-catching hologram pattern.
Manufacturer Web site: *www.learningcurve.com*

- Musical Take-Along Arch by Tiny Love
A tap of baby's hand, anywhere on the arch, will set off one of three playful tunes. Baby will love the instant feedback as she plays with the toys.
Manufacturer Web site: *www.tinylove.com*

- On-the-Go Musical Mobile by Tiny Love
With this toy, baby can enjoy the benefits of a crib mobile outside the crib. This portable musical mobile can be attached just about any-where to keep your baby entertained. The music, colors, and turning movement of the mobile will stimulate your baby's senses. The mobile features a lovely tune and three adorable flying bugs.
Manufacturer Web site: *www.tinylove.com*

- Tagalong Chimes by Infantino
Fascinate baby with the melody of chimes. These go-anywhere chime pals with convenient magnetic fasteners are perfect for car seats and stroller canopies.
Manufacturer Web site: *www.infantino.com*

- Take-Along Arch by Tiny Love
This arch features a set of bright colored, adorable, soft first toys. A bee with crinkly wings, a colorful mirror toy, and an adorable musical snail dangle from the toy bar.
Manufacturer Web site: *www.tinylove.com*

Rattles contribute to baby's early development. Playing with rattles provides her with a variety of stimulation throughout the day. Rattles come in different shapes, sizes, colors, and textures for babies to explore. Some rattles crinkle and jingle, while others play soft music. Rattles are wonderful for keeping little hands busy, and for relieving discomfort for teething babies.

○ Rattles

- Caterpillar Ring Rattle by Baby Einstein
  A brightly colored plush caterpillar wraps around this clear ring rattle. The center plastic bar holds three colorful textured rings, while the clear ring rattle contains brightly colored beads.
  Manufacturer Web site: *www.babyeinstein.com*

- Clarified Circle Rattle by Sassy
  Bright patterns and colors, soft sounds, and chewy textures will capture baby's imagination and stimulate her senses.
  Manufacturer Web site: *www.sassybaby.com*

- Easy Grip Rattle by Infantino
  The Easy-Grip Rattle is just the right fit for little hands, and features bright beads that rattle and roll.
  Manufacturer Web site: *www.infantino.com*

- Flipper Gripper Rattle by Sassy
  The top of this rattle spins; the movements, colors, patterns, textures, and sounds entertain baby.
  Manufacturer Web site: *www.sassybaby.com*

- Laugh & Learn Learning Keys by Fisher Price
  Laugh & Learn Learning Keys will open up a world of fun. The orange key has a blue car that spins and clicks, with textured rollers for added fun. The green key has sliding beads and a yellow house with a spinning door. The blue key has rattling beads and a red boat that slides along on the waves. Sing-along songs relate to all three keys. Clip the keys anywhere for take-along fun.
  Manufacturer Web site: *www.fisher-price.com*

- Sand Fish Rattle by Infantino
  This cute little fish friend has a twisting tail, teether fins, and colorful rattling beads.
  Vendor Web sites: *www.babyant.com*; *www.kidsurplus.com*

- Skwish by Manhattan Baby
  The smooth-textured Skwish fascinates babies with its web of brightly colored rods, beads, and balls. Skwish it and squash it every which way and the Skwish always bounces back to its original shape.
  Manufacturer Web site: *www.manhattantoy.com*

- Smiley Face Rattle by Sassy
  Smiley Face Rattle has dancing eyes, a nose that beeps, a big smile, and rattling beads. A mirror on the back helps develop self-awareness.
  Manufacturer Web site: *www.sassybaby.com*

○ Wrist and Foot Rattles
  At about four months of age, babies discover their hands and feet. Their natural hand waving and kicking motions will become a source of nonstop entertainment. Baby-soft wrist rattles and foot finders make playing with hands and feet exciting and fun for babies. These rattles stimulate sight, hearing, and touch.

  - Foot Rattles by Infantino
    Choose the cute bear or bunny rabbit to kick-start the fun.
    Manufacturer Web site: *www.infantino.com*

  - Gardenbug Footfinder and Wrist Rattle Set by Learning Curve
    With this rattle, cute little bees and ladybugs make looking at baby's hands and feet intriguing.
    Manufacturer Web site: *www.learningcurve.com*

  - Happy Feet Rattles by Sassy
    These soft socks put a smile on baby's face—and feet! Your baby will be delighted by a smiley face and a rattling sound in each foot.
    Manufacturer Web site: *www.sassybaby.com*

  - Wrist Rattles by Infantino
    Baby's hands dance with sound and action with these playful zoo characters.
    Manufacturer Web site: *www.infantino.com*

  - Wrist Rattles by Sassy
    A pair of soft rattles made of velour fabric attach easily to baby's wrists or ankles with Velcro closures. Cute animals make different noises.
    Manufacturer Web site: *www.sassybaby.com*

TEETHING TOYS

Teething can start anywhere from four to eight months of age, and sprouting teeth can be a painful process. You can relieve some of the pain by giving your baby toys that are specially designed for teething. Chewing on a teething toy can be comforting. They are usually made of rubber or soft plastic, in two or three textures. Your child can explore the surfaces to find out which texture is the most soothing. Teething rattles can be fun to play with, too. Many come in bright colors and have noisemakers.

○ Teething Toys
  - Fingers & Toes Teether by Safety 1st
    Babies love to put things in their mouths, especially their own hands and feet! Fingers & Toes Teethers are big, soft, and munchy teethers

with easy-grip handles to hold, and large fingers and toes to munch on.
Manufacturer Web site: *www.safety1st.com*

- Giggle Ball by Infantino
  Giggle Ball is a fun and colorful rattle toy. It's easy to grasp, with soft tubes connect the parts of the toy to each other and are perfect for teething babies. Brightly colored beads move back and forth, and the ball makes a fun giggle sound.
  Manufacturer Web site: *www.infantino.com*

- Gummy Guppy by Sassy
  Gummy Guppy has bumps, stars, ridges, and smooth areas for baby to explore and teethe on.
  Manufacturer Web site: *www.sassybaby.com*

- Link-a-Doos Teething Ring by Fisher Price
  This teething ring is easy to grasp and great for teething, with comforting beads sized just right. It's perfect for stimulating fun, with bright colors and interesting textures. And the easy-attach link keeps it in baby's hand and off of the floor.
  Manufacturer Web site: *www.fisher-price.com*

- Rings Around Rattle by Sassy
  This rattle has so much to watch, hear, and do; bright colors, rattling balls, sliding rings, and cushiony shapes give babies endless opportunities for creative exploration.
  Manufacturer Web site: *www.sassybaby.com*

- Springy Ringy by Sassy
  The Springy Ringy is a colorful, flexible teether that is easy to manipulate and provides lots of places for baby to place small hands. Baby can explore the shapes and textures with his mouth while teething.
  Manufacturer Web site: *www.sassybaby.com*

- Swim on the Rim Rattle by Sassy
  This lightweight rattle features a fish that sits on a clear plastic circle filled with brightly colored beads. Textured knobs encircle the plastic ring. The beads make a soft rattle sound, and the knobs are perfect for teething.
  Manufacturer Web site: *www.sassybaby.com*

○ Cool-Water-Filled Teething Toys
Cool-water-filled teethers help ease the pain and reduce the discomfort from swollen, sore gums. Place water-filled teethers in the refrigerator before you give them to your baby. Do not freeze teething toys or rings because the very cold temperature and hardness can hurt your baby's gums. It's a good idea to own several cool-water-filled teethers, so one will always be ready.

- Bumble Bites by Sassy
  This teething bee will keep baby busy. Each wing has a different texture for baby to explore with his mouth.
  Manufacturer Web site: *www.sassybaby.com*
- Caterpillar Cooling Teether by Baby Einstein
  This soft, water-filled teether has multiple textures with a brightly colored animated caterpillar handle that's easy for baby to grasp.
  Manufacturer Web site: *www.babyeinstein.com*
- Chilly Dilly Daisy by Sassy
  Chilly Dilly Daisy has a rattle in the center. Water-filled petals soothe aching gums while gripping, and textured petals are interesting to fingers.
  Manufacturer Web site: *www.sassybaby.com*
- Fun Ice Chewy Teethers by Munchkin
  Little fingers, toes, and baby chick have a textured surface and easy-to-grasp design that invites baby to bite and chew while the water's cooling action soothes tender gums.
  Manufacturer Web site: *www.munchkininc.com*
- Massaging Action Teether by The First Years
  This cool-water teether gently vibrates, massaging tender gums as soon as your child bites down.
  Manufacturer Web site: *www.thefirstyears.com*

This little star was the only toy that made my son feel better. The Massaging Action Teether is a must-have for any cranky teether!—Patricia

- Teething Tail Fish by Sassy
  This teether's brightly colored little fish, together with its many textured surfaces and water-filled fins, invite baby to soothe tender gums.
  Manufacturer Web site: *www.sassybaby.com*
- Teething Wing Butterfly by Sassy
  The Teething Wing Butterfly has one water-filled wing and one open wing for baby to grasp.
  Manufacturer Web site: *www.sassybaby.com*

HIGHCHAIR TOYS

Highchair toys are a great way to keep baby entertained while you're busy in the kitchen or preparing his meals. Place baby in his highchair with one of these cute toys, and he'll be entertained and won't mind the wait. If you have a fussy eater, the toys will divert his attention while you feed him. Some high-chair toys have a rubber suction cup base that makes them easy to attach to a highchair tray or table, or to a stroller with a tray. When they're not attached to a highchair, these toys can be used as rattles. Because eating can be quite a messy experience, you'll want to clean toys in warm soapy water and rinse them well after every meal.

○ Highchair Toys

- Fascination Station by Sassy
  Fascination Station is two toys in one. Used as a highchair toy, it spins, it flips, and it rattles. Then detach the toy from its suction-cup base, and it becomes an entertaining rattle.
  Manufacturer Web site: *www.sassybaby.com*

- Highchair Funny Farm by Infantino
  A cuddly cow, a crinkly chicken, and a pink, puffy pig keep baby company at mealtime.
  Vendor Web sites: *www.babycatalog.com*; *www.kidsurplus.com*

- Rocking Horse Rattle by Sassy
  The rocking horse rocks back and forth and can even turn somersaults on its stand. Colorful beads inside the horse's rocker make sounds whenever the rocking horse moves.
  Manufacturer Web site: *www.sassybaby.com*

- Rolling Ball by Graco
  Encourage developmental play from your little one with this fun and involving Rolling Ball toy. When baby hits the ball, the beads spin around, much to his delight. You will also find other suction-cup toys to choose from at this Web site.
  Manufacturer Web site: *www.gracobaby.com*

CAR-SEAT TOYS

Sitting in the back seat with nothing to do can get pretty boring. Car-seat toys are great for keeping baby busy in the car so Mom and Dad can concentrate on the road. Not only will these toys entertain your baby, they will also help develop her senses and imagination.

○ Car-Seat Toys

- 2-in-1 Traveling Guppy by Learning Curve
  This toy offers back seat fun for rear-facing and front-facing babies in car seats. Bright colors, contrasting patterns, and smiling faces attract your newborn's gaze. Jingling baby fish and a spinning see-through ball with rattling beads keep baby entertained while riding along.
  Manufacturer Web site: *www.learningcurve.com*

- Aqua Seal Kicker by Tiny Love
  A captivating cause-and-effect kick toy for the car, this toy has lights, music, and a soft aquarium with bubble action to keep baby busy.
  Manufacturer Web site: *www.tinylove.com*

- Barn Babies by Infantino
  The set includes a baby pig, rooster, and cow. Soft and easy to grasp, the animals squeak, rattle, and flutter to your child's content. Each brightly colored farm friend sports an attached nubby teething ring, and a clip-on link attaches to your stroller or car seat for take-along fun.
  Manufacturer Web site: *www.infantino.com*

- Link-a-Doos Car Seat Dashboard with Remote Control by Fisher Price
  The dashboard fits on baby's car seat and offers a selection of songs, lights, and activities to make outings more fun for both baby and you. You can use the remote control to activate either soothing or entertaining settings right from the driver's seat, or let baby start the fun.
  Manufacturer Web site: *www.fisher-price.com*

- Car Seat Gallery by Manhattan Baby
  Ten reversible cards with both black-and-white and color graphics help babies discover light/dark contrast and begin recognizing patterns. Hook-and-loop strap easily attaches to either front- or rear-facing car seats.
  Manufacturer Web site: *www.manhattanbaby.com*

- Clip & Go Musical Mobile by Tiny Love
  This musical mobile built for mobility fits most infant car seats, baby carriers, strollers, and cradles. It plays five continuous classical music tunes and also has a mute feature for silent visual stimulation.
  Manufacturer Web site: *www.tinylove.com*

- Developmental Travel Mobile by Sassy
  The Developmental Travel Mobile attaches to the back seat of automobiles. Characters are decorated in bold contrasting colors of black, white, and red. Each character makes rattle, chime, or jingle sounds and can be removed for attachment to your infant carrier or stroller.
  Manufacturer Web site: *www.sassybaby.com*

- Super Car Bar by Tiny Love
  The Super Car Bar is the ultimate car-seat toy. It has a padded steering wheel that turns, a play phone, an airplane that moves back and forth on a rail, and a diverse range of sounds to captivate baby's attention.
  Manufacturer Web site: *www.tinylove.com*

- Traveling Mobile by Lamaze
  The three detachable characters that rattle on this mobile are soft and cuddly—great for holding and hugging. The mobile will attach anywhere with its strong magnetic clasp.
  Manufacturer Web site: *www.learningcurve.com*

Keep baby entertained by attaching colorful toys to the stroller. Whether it's a toy bar, rattle, or mobile, it's sure to make the stroller ride more enjoyable.

○ Stroller Toys

- Busy Bug Bar by Sassy
  This toy's five fun activities keep baby entertained: a clicking flower, a spinning bee, a twirling beetle, a crinkling butterfly, and a cute bug cup to hold snacks.
  Manufacturer Web site: *www.sassybaby.com*

- Soft Stroller Bar by Sassy
  Soft Stroller Bar features a tethered caterpillar with antennas that light up, a baby snail that giggles, and a frog inside a book that ribbits. Pull the dragonfly to see it shake, rattle, and make a "buzzing" noise. Turtle-shaped snack cup is removable for easy cleaning.
  Manufacturer Web site: *www.sassybaby.com*

- Stroller Play Set by Tiny Love
  This set of three individual and unique activity toys includes a detachable honking horn with pull teethers, a soft baby chick that rattles and flips over, and colorful sliding beads. The detachable toys can be rearranged on the stroller bar to hold baby's interest—it's like having a new set of toys each time.
  Manufacturer Web site: *www.tinylove.com*

Your baby will play with activity gyms and arches starting at six weeks to eight weeks of age and continuing through his toddler months. Sight, sound, and motor stimulation are all important for baby's developing abilities. Many gyms have music and lights to keep your little one engaged in interactive play. Most arches are portable, so you can take them with you when you're traveling.

○ Musical Gyms

- Baby Gymtastics 3-in-1 Rockin Gym by Fisher Price
  Baby Gymtastics 3-in-1 Rockin Gym is a floor gym, a musical rocker, and take-along musical fun all in one. When baby is in the reclining position, the overhead gym plays music to an entertaining light show, with toys for baby to reach and bat. When baby gets older, you can easily convert the gym to a ride-on rocker that rewards movement with lively music and dancing lights. The xylophone keyboard detaches.
  Manufacturer Web site: *www.fisher-price.com*

- Classical Chorus Singing Stars Gym by Fisher Price
  Introduce your baby to classical music and children's songs with this musical gym. The Singing Stars Gym offers fascinating rewards from baby's

earliest days of reaching, through the sitting and playing stage, right up to when she's a toddler who loves to stand and play the piano keys. Manufacturer Web site: *www.fisher-price.com*

- Baby Playzone Kick & Whirl Carnival by Fisher Price
  A musical Ferris wheel on this toy rewards baby for kicking, reaching, and sitting. The overhead gym converts to a sit-up-and-play center as baby grows. Both are packed full of fun, with a ball-drop activity station, dancing lights, five minutes of lively music, spinners, ball ramps, and more. Manufacturer Web site: *www.fisher-price.com*

- Leapstart Gym by LeapFrog
  This two-stage gym features music, lights, foreign-language sounds, and learning. Hands-on activities help develop fine motor skills and encourage baby to reach and explore. For babies lying down, the gym is a multilearning experience with twinkling lights, instrumental melodies from around the world, and a motorized mobile. As your baby grows, the gym transforms to a sit-up activity center that introduces animal names, colors, and the numbers one through five in five languages. Manufacturer Web site: *www.leapfrog.com*

- Motion and Music Barnyard Gym by Fisher Price
  With motion, music, high-contrast patterns, and bright faces, this colorful gym is a great way to spark the senses. Baby bats at toys overhead to make a cow rock back and forth to delightful music and fun animal sounds. The youngest babies will enjoy the easy-to-reach side activities, with cute characters and a mirror for baby to reflect in, and sounds and textures to explore. Manufacturer Web site: *www.fisher-price.com*

○ Musical Play Arches with Play Mats
These musical play arches come with attachable play mats so you always have a clean surface for baby to lie on.

- Discover & Play Activity Gym by Baby Einstein
  The Discover & Play Activity Gym is a soft play gym with fun Baby Einstein characters on the mat that correspond with hanging plush characters. Toys include a star with lights. Press the center of the star and listen to classical music from Beethoven and Bach as you watch lights dance to the music. Other toys include plush characters that rattle, crinkle, and squeak, a soft book with animal pictures, and a baby-safe mirror. Manufacturer Web site: *www.babyeinstein.com*

- Discovering Water Activity Gym by Baby Einstein
  This colorful and entertaining gym includes a removable pat mat and a water-filled musical aquarium that plays six classical melodies and features dancing lights. Baby can watch the ocean animals swim inside both the aquarium and the pat mat. Baby will also love discovering the

real-world sea creatures underneath the peek-a-boo flaps and on the trilingual plastic discovery cards. This ocean environment also includes a plush Baby Neptune toy, a star-shaped mirror, and a prop-up pillow perfect for tummy-time play.
Manufacturer Web site: *www.babyeinstein.com*

- Gymini Super Deluxe Lights & Music by Tiny Love
  This Gymini features the Lights & Music Touch Pad, with classical music by Mozart and favorite nursery tunes to delight baby, with accompanying flashing lights. Whether on his tummy or his back, your baby will never get bored with the many toys and activities in this product.
  Manufacturer Web site: *www.tinylove.com*

- Gymini Total Playground—Kick & Play by Tiny Love
  The Gymini Total Playground offers a multisensory play experience, with a variety of sounds and images on the blanket and hanging toys, along with varied sensory stimulation provided by the different fabrics, textures, and shapes. The open/closed side border offers security for a small baby when the sides are up, and more play area when the sides are down for an older baby.
  Manufacturer Web site: *www.tinylove.com*

My son loves to kick, and this Gymini Total Playground is the best. There is so much for him to do on his back as well as for tummy time. I love how it folds for travel. It washes easily, too!—Carla

- Miracles & Milestones Magical Mobile Gym by Fisher Price
  Baby can lie on the comfortable panda mat and gaze up at the mobile with its large-view mirror, moving toys, and gently tracking lights. A combination of classical music and sung lullabies invites baby to listen. For tummy-time fun, remove the toys from the gym and place them on the floor where baby can reach and grab them.
  Manufacturer Web site: *www.fisher-price.com*

- Ocean Wonders Rockin' Aquarium Gym by Fisher Price
  With this toy, baby's batting or kicking at toys activates lights, five tunes, and three aquatic sounds, plus underwater movement in the "aquarium" on the toy bar. When baby's ready to sit up, the toy bar swings down, and the "aquarium" becomes a steering wheel. The unit includes removable fishy friends with rattle and jingle ball, lobster, and fish teethers.
  Manufacturer Web site: *www.fisher-price.com*

○ Nonmusical Play Arches and Gyms
Choose from these play arches and gyms without music but still chock full of fun activities and features.

- Entertain Me Play Gym by Boppy
  The Entertain Me Play Gym features a fabric mat and a boppy pillow for playtime comfort and support. Toys include a plush butterfly with lights and music, bee with crinkle wings, adjustable fabric baby-safe mirror, and water-filled ladybug. Five links attach toys to pillow, pad, or bars.
  Manufacturer Web site: *www.boppy.com*

- Gymini Deluxe Activity Gym by Tiny Love
  The Gymini Deluxe is a great travel toy. Toys dangle at varying heights for baby to enjoy while he's lying on his back or tummy. For traveling, just fold up the Gymini and carry it over your shoulder like a shoulder bag. When it's time to store the gym, return it to the special carrying case.
  Manufacturer Web site: *www.tinylove.com*

- Happy Hippo Gym by Infantino
  Whether it's playtime or naptime, the Happy Hippo Gym will keep baby entertained all day long! The padded playmat comes with extra support for baby's head and neck, as well as toys that include a plush bumblebee, musical flower, and dangling mirror. The removable activity arch easily attaches to cribs, and the convenient zip-up carrying case makes it the perfect travel gym for baby on the go.
  Manufacturer Web site: *www.infantino.com*

- Link-a-Doos Safari Activity Gym by Fisher Price
  With this toy, baby can rattle the zebra, crinkle the elephant, play peek-a-boo in the lion's mirror, or simply enjoy the bright colors and different textures. All of the linkable toys are detachable.
  Manufacturer Web site: *www.fisher-price.com*

ENTERTAINING TOYS

Babies love anything that moves, makes music, and has flashing lights.

○ Entertaining Toys

- Classical Keys by Sassy
  Here's a little piano sized just right for baby. Push on the keys and hear one of three classical music selections from Beethoven and Mozart. Watch the keys light up as the music plays. Two large, colorful beads slide around on the baby-grand-shaped handle for added play.
  Manufacturer Web site: *www.sassybaby.com*

- Movers & Shakers Zoo Friends by Infantino
  Babies have a blast watching the zoo animals scoot across the floor.
  Manufacturer Web site: *www.infantino.com*

- Ocean Wonders Musical Stacker by Fisher Price
  Baby can sort and stack the soft ocean friends on the post of this toy, or bat at the base to activate flashing goldfish lights and two different ocean-themed songs and sounds. The stackable ocean characters have lots of different textures, bright colors, and teethable areas.
  Manufacturer Web site: *www.fisher-price.com*

- Rolling Giggle Pals by The First Years
  Silly sounds reward baby's actions; a giggly puppy and giggly duck encourage baby's first grasps. Shake or roll the pals, and they laugh and bark or quack.
  Manufacturer Web site: *www.thefirstyears.com*

- Silly Sounds Television Remote by Sassy
  Baby can activate silly, cartoon-like sounds with the push of a button with this TV remote. The picture on the remote changes when it's moved back and forth, and the prism on top looks like the light changing on a real television remote.
  Manufacturer Web site: *www.sassybaby.com*

- Spiral Spin Top by Infantino
  Spinning balls and spiraling colors on this top are specially designed to fascinate baby. Simply press the top to watch the brightly colored balls spiral their way up the ramp and back down again.
  Manufacturer Web site: *www.infantino.com*

- Wiggles by The First Years
  Pull his tail, and he wiggles forward. Hold him and feel him vibrate. Hear the jingling sound effects and feel the variety of fabric textures.
  Manufacturer Web site: *www.thefirstyears.com*

○ Toy Accessories
- Lively Links by Sassy
  You can attach Lively Links to baby's highchair, car seat, or stroller.
  Manufacturer Web site: *www.sassybaby.com*

- Secure-a-Toy by Baby Buddy
  This clip-on strap keeps baby's toys and teethers close at hand, preventing them from being dropped or misplaced.
  Manufacturer Web site: *www.babybuddy.com*

- Tiny Love Rings by Tiny Love
  Tiny Love Rings are handy to have around. With them, you can hang toys on cribs, playpens, strollers, and more.
  Manufacturer Web site: *www.tinylove.com*

Reading to young children, even babies, encourages creative-thinking skills, promotes reading as an enjoyable activity, helps children develop mentally, gives them an appreciation for books, enhances their language and vocabulary development, and allows for quality family time. Find them at *www.amazon .com* or *www.bn.com*.

○ Baby's First Books

- Elmo's Busy Baby Book
  Author: Stephanie St. Pierre; Publisher: Random House, October 1999
  This book features Elmo and other babies from Sesame Street playing games such as peek-a-boo and patty-cake, and also has a noise-making toy bar across the front cover. It has a clackety dial, a squeaking push button, and other fun gadgets for baby's little fingers to explore.

- Goodnight Moon
  Author: Margaret Wise Brown; Publisher: HarperTrophy, January 2006
  This classic bedtime story, which has lulled generations of children to sleep, is the perfect first book to share with a child. Your child will say goodnight to all the objects in the book and add some goodnights to those special things of his own.

- Guess How Much I Love You
  Author: Sam McBratney; Publisher: Candlewick Press, May 2003
  During a bedtime game, every time Little Nutbrown Hare demonstrates how much he loves his father, Big Nutbrown Hare gently shows him that the love is returned even more.

- Pat the Bunny
  Author: Dorothy Kunhardt; Publisher: Golden Books, May 2001
  Babies love to touch and feel textures. This book takes your baby through a hands-on journey playing peek-a-boo, touching daddy's scratchy face, and more.

- Touch and Feel: Puppy
  Author: DK Preschool, March 1999
  Bright colors and touchable textures let baby see and feel the little puppies on the pages of this book. Baby will feel the puppy's fluffy tummy, silky ears, leathery nose, and other interesting textures.

- Where Is Baby's Belly Button?
  Author: Karen Katz; Publisher: Simon & Schuster, September 2000
  In this clever, multicultural peek-a-boo board book, babies can lift the flap and find the answers to questions like "Where are your eyes?" "Where are your hands?" and more.

Chapter 25
Master Shopping List for Part Two

This shopping list contains every product described in the preceding chapters. Once you've selected the products you wish to purchase, write in the brand names on the lines below. Bring this list with you on shopping trips, and check off each item as you make your purchases. You'll find these products at most department stores, discount stores, baby specialty shops, and online retailers. The numbers in parentheses designate the quantities of an item you'll need for a single baby, twins, or triplets, respectively. Where there are no numbers, just purchase as many as you feel you'll need.

CHAPTER 11: NEWBORN NECESSITIES

Diapers and Diaper Accessories

○ Pre-Folded or Flat Cloth Diapers
(4 doz.) (6 doz.) (8 doz.) _____

○ Cloth Diapers with Velcro Tabs
(4 doz.) (6 doz.) (8 doz.) _____

○ All-in-One-Style Diapers
(4 doz.) (6 doz.) (8 doz.) _____

○ Diaper Covers or Wraps (10) (12) (16) _____

○ Plastic Pants (8) (12) (18) _____

○ Diaper Pins (2 sets) (4 sets) (6 sets) _____

○ Disposable Preemie Diapers
(6 pkgs.) (12 pkgs.) (16 pkgs.) _____

○ Disposable Diapers (6 pkgs.) (12 pkgs.) (16 pkgs.) _____

Newborn Layette

○ Bodysuits or Onesies (5) (8) (12) _____

○ Gowns (5) (8) (12) _____

○ Footed Rompers or Sleep N Plays (5) (10) (15) _____

○ Sleep Sacks (2) (4) (6) _____

○ Blanket Sleepers (2) (4) (6) _____

○ Newborn Pairs of Booties or Socks (4) (8) (12) _____

○ Sweaters (2) (4) (6) _____

○ Newborn Hats (2) (4) (6) _____

○ Bibs (8) (12) (16) _____

○ Receiving Blankets (6) (12) (15) _____

○ Easy Wrap Swaddler (6) (12) (15) _____

○ Burp Cloths (2 doz.) (3 doz.) (3 doz.) _____

○ Lap Pads (9) (12) (15) _____

○ Changing-Table Pad Covers (2) (3) (3) _____

○ Hooded Bath Towels (2) (4) (6) _____

○ Washcloths (6) (12) (15) _____

○ Preemie Clothing _____

Crib Bedding

- ⭕ Crib Mattress—Foam or Coil (1) (2) (3) _____
- ⭕ Fitted Waterproof or Quilted Mattress Pads (2) (4) (6) _____
- ⭕ Fitted Crib Sheets (2) (4) (6) _____
- ⭕ Crib Blankets (2) (4) (6) _____
- ⭕ Bumper Pads (1) (2) (3) _____
- ⭕ Special Bumper Pads (1) (2) (3) _____
- ⭕ Traditional Crib Bumpers (1) (2) (3) _____
- ⭕ Complete Crib Bedding Sets (1) (2) (3) _____

Bassinet Bedding

- ⭕ Bassinet Pads (1) (2) (3) _____
- ⭕ Bassinet Bumper (1) (2) (3) _____
- ⭕ Bassinet Mattress Pad Covers (2) (4) (6) _____
- ⭕ Bassinet Sheets (2) (4) (6) _____
- ⭕ Complete Bassinet Bedding Sets (1) (2) (3) _____

Cradle Bedding

- ⭕ Cradle Pad (1) (2) (3) _____
- ⭕ Cradle Mattress Pad Covers (2) (4) (6) _____
- ⭕ Cradle Bumpers (1) (2) (3) _____
- ⭕ Cradle Sheets (2) (4) (6) _____
- ⭕ Complete Cradle Bedding Sets (1) (2) (3) _____

Inserts for Parents' Bed

- ⭕ Baby Bed Inserts for Parent's Bed (1)—
  only big enough for a single baby _____

CHAPTER 12: NURSERY FURNITURE

- ⭕ Crib (1) (2) (3) _____
- ⭕ Changing Table _____

CHAPTER 12: NURSERY FURNITURE (continued)

- ⭕ Dresser (I) or (2), depending on your needs _____
- ⭕ Glider Rocker_____
- ⭕ Ottoman_____
- ⭕ Small Table _____
- ⭕ Arm's Reach Bedside Co-Sleeper
  (I) for as many as triplets _____
- ⭕ Leg Extensions (I set per co-sleeper) _____
- ⭕ Arm's Reach Co-Sleeper Netting _____
- ⭕ Arm's Reach Co-Sleeper Canopy _____
- ⭕ Co-Sleeper Fitted Sheets (2 per co-sleeper) _____
- ⭕ Arm's Reach Co-Sleeper Floor Length Liner _____

CHAPTER 13: NURSERY NECESSITIES

- ⭕ Pacifiers (3) (6) (9) _____
- ⭕ Preemie Pacifiers (3) (6) (9) _____
- ⭕ Diaper Pail _____
- ⭕ Diaper Wipes Warmer _____
- ⭕ Sleep Positioners (I) (2) (3)_____
- ⭕ Baby Monitor (I, with two receivers)_____
- ⭕ Sounds and Movement Monitor (I per crib) _____
- ⭕ Video Monitor_____
- ⭕ Hamper_____
- ⭕ Wastebasket _____
- ⭕ Lamp (I) or (2), as needed _____
- ⭕ Clock_____
- ⭕ Night Light _____
- ⭕ Hangers_____
- ⭕ Combination Smoke and Carbon Monoxide Detector _____

CHAPTER 14: NURSERY NICETIES

- ○ Bassinet_____
- ○ Cradle_____
- ○ Moses Basket_____
- ○ Mobile—Battery Operated_____
- ○ Mobile—Suction Cup, Wall Mounted_____
- ○ Changing-Table Mobile_____
- ○ Diaper and Diaper Wipes Holder_____
- ○ Diaper Stacker_____
- ○ Elevated Sleep Positioner (1) (2) (3)_____
- ○ Nature Sounds and Lullaby Player_____
- ○ Cassette Player_____
- ○ Scale_____
- ○ Dreft Laundry Soap_____
- ○ Stain and Odor Remover and Prewash_____

CHAPTER 15: NURSERY ACCESSORIES

- ○ Scented Drawer Liners_____
- ○ Closet Organizers_____
- ○ Pictures and Wall Hangings_____
- ○ Door Plaques_____
- ○ Growth Charts (1) (2) (3)_____
- ○ Bookends_____
- ○ Children's Knobs and Drawer Pulls_____
- ○ Switch Plates_____

CHAPTER 16: KEEPSAKES

- ○ Hand-Print Set_____
- ○ Picture Frames_____
- ○ Piggy Bank_____
- ○ Keepsake Box_____

Bathtubs and Bath Seats

○ Baby Bathtub _____

○ Bath Seat _____

Bath-Time Cleansing Products

○ Baby Bath Soap _____

○ All-in-One Body Wash and Shampoo _____

○ Vapor Bath _____

○ Shampoo _____

○ Cradle-Cap Shampoo _____

Grooming Products

○ Brush and Comb Set _____

○ Baby Nail Scissors _____

○ Baby Nail Clippers_____

○ Emery Boards _____

○ Complete Manicure Set_____

○ Complete Grooming Set _____

○ Combination Grooming and Health-Care Kit _____

Bath-Time Accessories

○ Tub-Side Knee and Elbow Savers for Parents_____

○ Spray Attachment for Bath or Sink_____

○ Bath Visor_____

○ Toy Bag _____

○ Digital Thermometer _____

○ Nasal Aspirator _____

○ Infant Saline Nose Drops _____

○ Cotton Swabs _____

○ Rubbing Alcohol _____

○ Small Jar of Petroleum Jelly _____

○ 2-inch x 2-inch Sterile Gauze Pads _____

○ Calibrated Medication Dispenser _____

○ Fever Reducer _____

○ Gas-Relief Drops _____

○ Infant Glycerin Suppositories _____

○ Teething Gel _____

○ Vaporizer _____

○ Humidifier _____

○ Health-Care Kit _____

CHAPTER 19: SKIN-CARE PRODUCTS

○ Non-Allergenic Diaper Wipes _____

○ Diaper Rash Creams and Ointments _____

○ Baby Lotion _____

○ Sunscreen Lotions or Spray _____

○ Sunblock Stick _____

○ Soothing Product for Dry or Sunburned Skin _____

CHAPTER 20: PRODUCTS FOR NURSING MOTHERS

Breast Pumps

○ Top-of-the-Line Electric Breast Pumps _____

○ Mini Electric Breast Pumps _____

○ Manual Breast Pumps _____

Breast Pumps

○ Extra Breast Shield System _____

○ Extra Valve/Membrane Assembly _____

○ Extra Tubing_____

○ Breast Milk Collection and Storage Bags _____

○ Storage Clips and Labels _____

○ Cleaning Products _____

  ● Cavacide—Germicidal Cleaner

  ● Quick Clean Micro Steam Bags

○ Vehicle Lighter Adapter _____

Nursing Comfort

○ Nursing Pads _____

  ● Washable Nursing Pads

  ● Disposable Nursing Pads

○ Nipple Lotions and Creams_____

○ Breast Therapy Warm/Cold Packs_____

○ Breast Shells_____

○ Nipple Shields _____

○ Inverted Nipple Products _____

○ Nursing Stool _____

○ Nursing Pillow _____

○ Nursing Pillow for Twins_____

○ Nursing Bibs_____

Other Nursing Accessories

○ Nursing Breast Pad Case _____

○ Nursing Pillow Covers _____

○ Hands-Free Pumping Attachments _____

○ Bottles (12) (24) (30) _____

  ● Reusable Bottles

  ● Disposable Bottles

○ Nipples (12) (24) (30) _____

○ Hands-Free Bottle Systems (1) (2) (3) _____

  ● Hands-Free Baby Feeding System

  ● Pacifeeder

Bottle and Nipple Accessories

○ Bottle and Nipple Brush (1) (2) (3) _____

○ Dishwasher Basket for Nipples, Rings, Caps, and Pacifiers
  (1) (2) (2) _____

○ Drying Rack for Bottles, Nipples, Rings, Caps, and Pacifiers
  (1) (2) (2) _____

○ Sterilizer _____

○ Bottle Warmer (1) (2) (2) _____

○ Baby Bottle and Food Carousels_____

Powdered Formula

○ Powdered Formula _____

○ 64-Ounce Calibrated Measuring Cup _____

○ One-Cup Calibrated Measuring Cup_____

○ Wire Whisk _____

Feeding Accessories

○ Temperature-Sensitive Feeding Spoons_____

○ Feeding Spoons Without a Temperature-Sensitive Safety Tip_____

○ Feeding Bowls with Suction-Cup Base_____

○ Food Processor _____

○ Hands-Free Baby-Bottle Holders (1) (2) (3) _____

  ● The Bottle Bundle

Exercising Equipment

○ Exersaucer (1) (2) (3) _____

○ Doorway Jumper (1) (2) (3) _____

○ Floor Jumper (1) (2) (3) _____

Swings and Swing Accessory

○ Standard Swing (1) (2) (3) _____

○ Cradle Swing (1) (2) (3) _____

○ Travel Swing (1) (2) (3) _____

Bouncy Seats and Bouncy Bassinet

○ Bouncy Seat with Vibration (1) (2) (3) _____

○ Bouncy Bassinet_____

High Chair and High-Chair Accessories

○ Highchair (1) (2) (3) _____

- Highchair Activity Tray (1) (2) (3)
- Prima Pappa Dinner Tray (1) (2) (3)
- Secure-a-Toy (1) (2) (3)
- Sesame Street Meal & Play Mat (1) (2) (3)

Portable Hook-On High Chairs and Booster Seats

○ Portable Hook-On Highchair (1) (2) (3) _____

○ Portable Booster Seat (1) (2) (3) _____

○ Inflatable Portable Booster Seat (1) (2) (3) _____

Pack 'N Playard and Pack 'N Play Accessories

○ Pack 'N Play Playard _____

- Pack 'N Play Pads (1 for every Pack 'N Play)
- Pack 'N Play Sheets (2 for every Pack 'N Play)
- Pack 'N Play Netting (1 for every Pack 'N Play)
- Pack 'N Play Changing Table Pad Cover (2 for every Pack 'N Play)

- Pack 'N Play Canopy (1 for every Pack 'N Play)
- Pack 'N Play Playard Diaper Organizer (1 for every Pack 'N Play)
- Pack 'N Play Tent Plus Cabana Kit (1 for every Pack 'N Play)
- Pack 'N Play Twins Playard Sheets (2 for every Pack 'N Play)
- Pack 'N Play Playard Electronics Unit (1 for every Pack 'N Play)

Standard Playpen

○ Playpen _____

Stroller for a Single Baby

○ Umbrella Stroller_____

○ Lightweight Stroller_____

○ Standard Stroller _____

○ Travel System_____

○ Jogging-Stroller Travel System _____

○ Snap-N-Go Stroller _____

○ Jogging Stroller_____

○ Carriage or Pram_____

○ Tandem Stroller with Stadium Seating_____

Strollers for Multiples

○ Twin Side-by-Side Stroller _____

○ Twin Tandem Stroller_____

○ Twin Jogging Stroller_____

○ Triplet Side-by-Side Stroller_____

○ Triplet Tandem Stroller_____

○ Triplet Jogging Stroller _____

○ Quad Side-by-Side Stroller _____

○ Quad Tandem Stroller _____

○ Snap-N-Go Stroller _____

Stroller Accessories

○ Single Stroller Rain Shield_____

○ Twin Side-by-Side Stroller Rain Shield _____

○ Twin Tandem Stroller Rain Shield_____

○ Jogging Stroller Rain Shield_____

○ Single Stroller Netting_____

○ Twin Stroller Netting _____

○ Single Jogging Stroller Netting_____

○ Double Jogging Stroller Netting _____

○ Single Stroller Sunshade _____

○ Double Stroller Sunshade _____

○ Stroller Organizer _____

○ Drink Holders _____

○ Snack Holders _____

○ Single Stroller Travel Bags _____

○ Twin Stroller Travel Bags _____

○ Umbrella Stroller Travel Bags _____

○ Stroller Seat Protectors _____

○ Stroller Umbrella_____

○ Stroller Blanket _____

○ Stroller Connector _____

○ Stroller Extension Handle _____

Car Seat (1) (2) (3)

○ Infant Car Seat/Carrier_____

○ Convertible Car Seat _____

○ Toddler/Booster Car Seat _____

Car Seat/Carrier Accessories

○ Infant Car-Seat Cover_____

○ Car-Seat Mirrors for Rear-Facing Car Seats _____

○ Car-Seat Mirrors for Front-Facing Car Seats_____

○ Sunshades_____

○ Head Support _____

○ Total Body Support_____

○ Car-Seat Strap Cover_____

○ Car-Seat Canopy_____

○ Car-Seat Bunting_____

○ Car-Seat Organizer_____

○ Car-Seat Protector _____

○ Car-Seat Shield _____

○ Car-Seat Mobile _____

○ Vehicle Upholstery Protector for Single Car Seat _____

○ Car-Seat Travel Bag_____

Infant Carriers

○ Sling_____

○ Front/Back Carrier _____

○ Infant Carrier for Multiples_____

○ Backpack Carrier_____

○ Stroller Backpack_____

CHAPTER 23: TRAVELING ACCESSORIES

○ Insulated Bottle and Food Bags_____

○ Extra Hot and Cool Gel Packs _____

○ Bottle Holder_____

○ Vehicle Adapter Bottle Warmer_____

○ Wraparound Bottle Warmer _____

○ Portable Food Bowl _____

○ Portable Changing Pad_____

○ Cloth Shopping-Cart Covers _____

○ Disposable Shopping-Cart Handle Covers _____

○ Portable Travel Bed _____

CHAPTER 24: TOYS FOR BABY'S FIRST YEAR

Baby's First Toys

○ Black, White, and Red Toys_____

Crib Toys

○ Plush Slumbertime Soothers_____

○ Musical Slumbertime Soothers _____

○ Musical Crib Toys _____

○ Soft Crib Toys _____

Crib Mirrors

○ Musical Crib Mirrors_____

○ Nonmusical Crib Mirrors_____

○ Musical Pull-String Toys _____

Bathtub Toys

○ Bobbing, Floating, Squirting Toys _____

Rattles

○ Hand-Held Rattles _____

○ Wrist and Foot Rattles_____

○ Teething Toys_____

○ Cool-Water-Filled Teething Toys _____

High-Chair Toys

○ Suction-Cup Toys _____

On-the-Go Toys

○ Infant Car-Seat/Carrier Toys _____

○ Car-Seat Toys_____

○ Stroller Toys_____

Activity Gyms and Arches

○ Musical Gyms_____

○ Musical Play Arches with Play Mats _____

○ Nonmusical Play Arches and Gyms _____

Entertaining Toys

○ Scooting Toys _____

○ Stacking Toys _____

○ Sound, Music, and Light Toys_____

Toy Accessories

○ Link-a-Doos 20-Link Pack _____

○ Lively Links_____

○ Secure-a-Toy _____

○ Tiny Love Rings Set_____

Baby's First Books

○ *Good Night Moon* _____

○ *Pat the Bunny* _____

○ *Guess How Much I Love You* _____

○ *Where Is Baby's Belly Button?* _____

○ *Elmo's Busy Baby Book*_____

Part Three

Books, Videos, DVDs, and Music

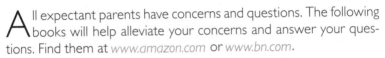

Chapter 26
Pregnancy Library

A ll expectant parents have concerns and questions. The following books will help alleviate your concerns and answer your questions. Find them at *www.amazon.com* or *www.bn.com*.

○ Pregnancy and Childbirth Books

- *Natural Childbirth the Bradley Way: Revised Edition*
  Author: Susan McCutcheon-Rosegg; Publisher: Plume, July 1996
  Since the Bradley method was first introduced in 1970, a growing number of expectant parents have opted for natural childbirth, knowing that it's safer than medicated or surgical delivery. This book provides all the answers, offering sound advice on how to prepare physically for labor and what to expect during each of its stages.

- *The Birth Book*
  Authors: William and Martha Sears; Publisher: Little, Brown and Company, February 1994
  William and Martha Sears, pediatric specialists, detail the options available to today's expectant parents in an up-to-date, factual, and unbiased fashion. This comprehensive, reassuring, and authoritative guide thoroughly explores the abundant choices couples face when they are anticipating the birth of their child.

- *The Complete Book of Pregnancy and Childbirth*
  Author: Shelia Kitzinger; Publisher: Alfred A. Knopf, December 2003
  Extensively revised to reflect recent scientific advances and cultural trends, this indispensable guide provides you with all the information you want to know about being pregnant and giving birth. The book includes sections on prenatal care, exercise, delivery methods, and baby's development in the uterus.

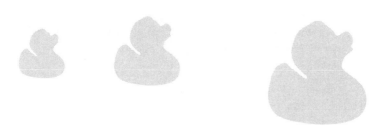

- *The Girlfriends' Guide to Pregnancy: Or Everything Your Doctor Won't Tell You*
  Author: Vicki Lovine; Publisher: Pocket, January 1997
  A delivery-room veteran gives you the lowdown as only a best friend can. From the top ten lies, such as, "Maternity clothes are so much cuter now," to the long-awaited birth, here are practical tips and hilarious takes on everything to do with being pregnant. Through this very popular book, Vicki Lovine helps you achieve a healthy and emotionally fulfilling pregnancy and childbirth.

I absolutely loved "The Girlfriends' Guide." Whenever I felt fat or depressed I would pick up the book and read a little. I would recommend this book to every pregnant woman with a good sense of humor.—Teresa

- *What to Expect When You're Expecting*
  Authors: Arlene Eisenberg, Heidi Murkoff, and Sandee Hathaway; Publisher: Workman Publishing Company, April 2002
  This popular guide offers expectant parents all the answers to their many questions. This attractively designed, month-by-month guide is divided into five sections that cover every stage of pregnancy, with places to note pregnancy tests, labor diary, and birth record.

○ Multiple-Birth Pregnancies

- *Double Duty: The Parents' Guide to Raising Twins from Pregnancy Through the School Years*
  Author: Christina Baglivi Tinglof; Publisher: McGraw-Hill, June 1998
  The author gives reassuring advice on a variety of topics such as having a healthy pregnancy, bed rest, breast versus bottle feeding, the pros and cons of dressing twins alike, setting up the nursery, developmental milestones, separate classrooms, staying home or returning to work, and much more.

- *Everything You Need to Know to Have a Healthy Twin Pregnancy*
  Authors: Gila Leiter and Rachel Krantz; Publisher: Dell Publishing Company, November 2000
  Dr. Leiter, a mother of twins, takes you step-by-step through the processes of pregnancy and birth. She and Krantz provide answers to all your questions, plus practical know-how, psychological support, and extensive resources for this most joyous and overwhelming experience, whether you're having two babies or four.

- *Keys to Parenting Multiples*
  Authors: Karen Kerkhoff Gromada and Mary C. Hurlburt; Publisher: Barron's Educational Series, February 2001
  Designed to be both a quick read and an easy reference, this guide features forty-five brief chapters so parents can find just the information they're seeking. Chapters on decreasing risks while carrying twins, products, breastfeeding, household organization, naming, bonding, and finding the support you need can help expectant or new parents surmount the sometimes overwhelming feelings they might experience when they know they're having multiples.

- *The Multiple Pregnancy Sourcebook: Pregnancy and the First Days with Twins, Triplets, and More*
  Author: Nancy Bowers, RN; Publisher: McGraw-Hill, April 2001
  This book explores the physical, financial, and emotional challenges of this high-risk condition. All information is aimed specifically at multiple pregnancies. You'll find information on nutrition, routine visits, testing, actual labor, postnatal care, selective reduction, bed rest, and the chances of having at least one baby delivered by cesarean section.

- *When You're Expecting Twins, Triplets, or Quads, Revised Edition: Proven Guidelines for a Healthy Multiple Pregnancy*
  Authors: Barbara Luke and Tamara Eberlein; Publisher: Collins, June 2004
  Dr. Luke outlines a practical nutritional program to keep you and your babies healthy. She also offers a comprehensive tour of what you can expect during your unique pregnancy and childbirth. Subjects discussed in this book are nutrition, Mom's changing body and emotions,

fetal development, potential complications, bed rest, and labor and delivery.

○ Birth Partner

- *The Birth Partner, Second Edition: Everything You Need to Know to Help a Woman Through Childbirth*
  Author: Penny Simkin; Publisher: Harvard Common Press, June 2001
  Helping a woman through childbirth can be a daunting experience. No matter what your relation to the expectant mom, this book will help prepare you for every step of the birthing process.

○ Breastfeeding
Breastfeeding should be a relaxing and wonderful experience. Getting off to the right start is essential. These books are excellent guides to successfully breastfeeding your baby.

- *Nursing Mother's Companion*
  Author: Kathleen Huggins; Publisher: Harvard Common Press, March 2005
  This accessible guide covers what women need to know about breastfeeding. From topics such as breast pumps to going back to work to tips on finding a comfortable nursing position, this book gives sound advice on making breastfeeding approachable and satisfying for mother and child.

- *Nursing Mother's Guide to Weaning*
  Author: Kathleen Huggins; Publisher: Harvard Common Press, October 1994
  This book helps nursing mothers learn how to wean their children with as much love as they nursed them. Mothers will be able to recognize when both they and their children are ready to wean.

- *Nursing Mother, Working Mother*
  Author: Gale Pryor; Publisher: Harvard Common Press, February 1996
  Gayle Pryor helps you figure out how to manage the stresses of returning to work and how to optimize your nursing situation. She explains, clearly and thoroughly, everything a working mother needs to know, from breastfeeding and bonding basics to choosing a childcare provider. This book also touches on expressing and storing milk at work, and combating fatigue.

- *The Breastfeeding Book: Everything You Need to Know About Nursing Your Child from Birth Through Weaning*
  Authors: Martha and William Sears; Publisher: Little, Brown and Company, March 2000
  Taking a realistic, contemporary approach, Martha and William Sears bring an age-old practice completely up to date. Their encyclopedic guide to the art and science of breastfeeding enables all women to experience and enjoy one of nature's most rewarding relationships.

- *The Complete Book of Breastfeeding*
  Authors: Marvin S. Eiger, Sally Wendkos Olds, Wendy Wray, and Roe Di Bona; Publisher: Bantam, September 1999
  This is a wonderful guide with abundant information on a variety of topics related to breastfeeding. This book has lots of great tips on how to make breastfeeding easier and how to handle the possible problems you may encounter.

I love "The Complete Book of Breastfeeding"! As a first-time mother, I could not have been happier with the extensive explanations and information provided.—Katie

○ Books for Expectant Dads
  Fatherhood presents some of the greatest challenges and greatest opportunities men ever face. Along with the pleasure children can bring, they also create new demands and situations that help dads change and grow as people. The books listed in this section were written especially for expectant dads to help prepare them for fatherhood. These books explore pregnancy, birth, and child rearing, and they provide important support. New dads will learn how to change diapers, fix bottles, and soothe crying babies. Baby accomplishments important to new fathers, such as first sounds and movements, are explained in terms of child development. In addition, new fathers will learn how to develop important traits and skills such as patience, sensitivity, and communication.

  - *She's Had a Baby: And I'm Having a Meltdown*
    Author: James Douglas Barron; Publisher: Harper Paperbacks, June 1999
    This survival guide for dads offers guidance on making the challenge of fatherhood all it can be. Barron champions the joys and anxieties of daddyhood, while helping a man to cope with the ups and downs a relationship can go through during this time.

  - *The Expectant Father: Facts, Tips, and Advice for Dads-to-Be*
    Authors: Armin A. Brott and Jennifer Ash; Publisher: Abbeville Press, May 2001
    This book helps expectant fathers prepare for the big day and life at home with a new baby. It helps men feel more connected to their partner during those important months of pregnancy, understand the physical changes their partner is going through, and follow the baby's development.

  - *The Joy of Fatherhood: The First Twelve Months*
    Author: Marcus Jacob Goldman; Publisher: Three Rivers Press, May 2000

With scores of tips and pages of timely advice, this book is just the cure for the bewildered new father—or the perfect refresher for the experienced dad. *The Joy of Fatherhood* covers hundreds of topics, such as changing a diaper, bathing the baby, financial planning, and much more, and it includes a preparation checklist for the month before birth.

- *The New Father: A Dad's Guide to the First Year*
  Author: Armin A. Brott; Publisher: Abbeville Press, May 2004
  This book skillfully and humorously guides men through the daunting experience of being a new father, from birth through the toddler years. This informative book helps new dads feel better about their often confusing role. The book is arranged month by month, so dads can easily access the information they need right when they need it.

○ Baby Naming Books
Deciding on just the right name for your baby can be a complex and difficult task. You would be surprised at how much time and energy the process can take. Whether you're looking for a common name or a unique name, you're sure to find just the right one in one of these books.

- *Beyond Jennifer & Jason, Madison & Montana*
  Authors: Linda Rosenkrantz and Pamela Redmond Satranl; Publisher: St. Martin's Press, Inc., August 2006
  Beyond Jennifer & Jason, Madison & Montana uniquely identifies the trends, styles, and connotations in today's baby naming game.

- *The Everything Baby Names Book*
  Authors: Lisa Shaw, Lisa Rogak, and Lisa Angowski Shaw; Publisher: Adams Media Corp., January 1997
  Everything you need to know to pick the perfect name for your baby is covered in this book. It takes a fun look at choosing names and includes diverse name lists, such as the most popular names in each decade, the names of angels, characters from literature, world leaders, and more.

I found "The Everything Baby Names Book" to be just about everything I was looking for in a name book. It gave a wide variety of names along with their meanings and origins.—Heidi

- *The Greatest Baby Name Book Ever*
  Author: Carol McD. Wallace; Publisher: HarperCollins, July 2004
  Choose from literally thousand of names, from the traditional to the unique to the completely new and original, and find the one that's just

right for your baby. The history, meaning, and spelling variations of names are also discussed.

○ Pregnancy Journals
Keeping a journal is a good way to keep track of all that's going on during your pregnancy. You can keep a record of your feelings, thoughts, and dreams in any one of the journals listed here. If you have more than one child, you can compare pregnancies using your pregnancy journals.

- *The Pregnancy Journal: A Day-to-Day Guide to a Happy and Healthy Pregnancy*
  Author: A. Christine Harris; Publisher: Chronicle Books LLC, August 1996
  This keepsake book will inspire, encourage, and guide mothers-to-be to fill the pages with ideas and sketches. *The Pregnancy Journal* reassures mothers-to-be about their baby's developmental stages, and provides room to record thoughts, experiences, and the joys of pregnancy.

- *The What to Expect When You're Expecting Pregnancy Organizer*
  Authors: Arlene Eisenberg, Heidi Murkoff, and Sandee Hathaway; Publisher: Workman Publishing Company, January 1995
  This complete pregnancy organizer provides a place to record everything that occurs during your pregnancy. It includes five sections that make it easy to find what you need: "Prenatal Care," "Pregnancy Journal," "Getting Ready for Baby," "Getting Ready for Childbirth," and "Baby's Arrival."

- *Your Pregnancy Week-by-Week*
  Authors: Glade B. Curtis and Judith Schuler; Publisher: Da Capo Press, January 2004
  This is a keepsake journal to chart your progress and thoughts, packed with information for a safe and healthy pregnancy. This unique book is divided into each week of pregnancy, with important information about your developing baby and your changing body.

○ Prenatal Fitness
Many women are concerned about maintaining fitness during and after pregnancy. Exercising during pregnancy will improve your overall energy level and stamina; relieve discomfort; and improve posture, circulation, and digestion. Exercising can also help relieve tension and stress, and keep you emotionally balanced, which will help prepare you for labor and the delivery of your baby. These books will teach you how to implement an exercise program before you get pregnant, as well as how to safely continue exercising during and after your pregnancy. Before you start any exercise program, be sure to check with your doctor.

- *Denise Austin's Ultimate Pregnancy Book: How to Stay Fit and Healthy Through the Nine Months—And Shape Up After Baby*
  Author: Denise Austin; Publisher: Simon & Schuster, May 1999

This is a comprehensive guide that answers many common questions related to maintaining fitness during and after pregnancy, workout techniques, and nutritional needs, and offers advice about getting your body back in shape after baby is born.

- *Exercising Through Your Pregnancy*
  Author: James F. Clapp III; Publisher: Addicus Books, March 2002
  Dr. Clapp offers specific exercise recommendations for all stages of the pregnancy, from preconception to postdelivery. Learn how to implement an exercise program before you get pregnant, as well as how to safely continue exercising during and after your pregnancy.

This book is an excellent read for those who are serious about exercise and who are pregnant or thinking about becoming pregnant.—Jamie

- *Pregnancy Fitness: Mind Body Spirit*
  Author: Fitness Magazine with Ginny Graves; Publisher: Crown Publishing Group, August 1999
  Pregnancy Fitness, by the experts at *Fitness Magazine*, provides expectant mothers with all the information they need to exercise safely and effectively throughout their pregnancy. This book guides you carefully through every trimester, covering the physical changes and common complaints for each one, from shortness of breath to dizziness to morning sickness. Chapters on cardiovascular fitness and getting stronger help you develop the aerobic capacity and muscles to carry your growing child with greater comfort, and prepare you for labor. *Pregnancy Fitness* will help ensure a healthy pregnancy, an easy delivery, and a speedy recovery.

- *The Pilates Pregnancy: Maintaining Strength, Flexibility, and Your Figure*
  Authors: Mari Winsor and Mark Laska; Publisher: Perseus Publishing, November 2001
  A wonderful conditioning exercise for women of all shapes and sizes, Pilates is now recognized as one of the best overall exercises for the pregnant body, as well. Organized into workouts for each trimester, *The Pilates Pregnancy* shows expectant mothers how to increase flexibility and reduce stress during pregnancy, and so make getting back into shape after childbirth easier.

- Prenatal Yoga
  Pregnancy is exciting, but also physically stressful. Yoga provides an ideal way to prepare women for the many physical and emotional changes that

accompany pregnancy by using the quiet practice of gentle exercise. Yoga can bring a harmony to mind and body that has far-reaching effects during this important time. Pregnancy calls upon a woman's physical, mental, and emotional resources like no other life experience, and practicing yoga is an excellent way to remain strong and relaxed in all three ways.

- *Prenatal Yoga and Natural Childbirth*
  Author: Jeannine Parvati Baker; Publisher: North Atlantic Books, November 2001
  Featured are detailed, illustrated yoga instructions designed specifically for pregnant women; honest, down-to-earth accounts of the birth process; and information about birthing choices.

- *Step-by-Step Yoga for Pregnancy: Essential Exercises for the Childbearing Years*
  Author: Wendy Teasdill; Publisher: McGraw-Hill, April 2000
  Step-by-Step Yoga for Pregnancy is an essential guide to the best exercises for each stage of pregnancy, and to the resources you need for a harmonious pregnancy, birth, and recovery.

- *Yoga for Pregnancy, Birth, and Beyond*
  Author: Franciose Barbira Freedman; Publisher: DK Publishing Inc., June 2004
  Organized into two sections, this fully illustrated manual, designed for pregnant women at all levels of fitness and with no prior knowledge of yoga, provides a basic introduction to the technique, including proper breathing, postures, and relaxation methods. Easy-to-follow exercises are arranged in sequences for each trimester, and include labor and birthing positions.

- *Yoga for Pregnancy: Ninety-Two Safe, Gentle Stretches Appropriate for Pregnant Women and New Mothers*
  Author: Sandra Jordan; Publisher: St. Martin's Press, January 2005
  Yoga, with its emphasis on body awareness, breathing, and relaxation, is helping growing numbers of pregnant women adjust to the physical and mental demands of labor, birth, and motherhood. Provided here are ninety-two Iyengar poses carefully chosen as being safe and effective during and after pregnancy.

○ *Nutritional Fitness*
Proper prenatal nutrition is important to your health and the development of your baby. During pregnancy, what you eat can affect your weight, help prevent morning sickness, and affect your child's physical and emotional development.

- *Eating for Two: The Complete Guide to Nutrition During Pregnancy*
  Authors: Mary Abbott Hess, Anne Elise Hunt, and Roy M. Pitkin; Publisher: John Wiley & Sons, February 1991

This book was written for pregnant women who are concerned about getting proper nutrition during pregnancy, *Eating for Two* offers an eating program women can adapt to their tastes and needs. Topics covered include weight gain, vitamins, minerals, the effect diet has on fetal development, bottle versus breastfeeding, and more.

- *Every Woman's Guide to Eating During Pregnancy*
  Authors: Martha Rose Shulman, M.D., and Jane Davis; Publisher: Houghton Mifflin, August 2002
  Now that you're pregnant, what you eat is more important than ever before. You may be nauseous, starving, or alternately one or the other, and your tastes may change constantly. Whatever your condition, whether you're twenty-seven or forty-seven, and whether you love cooking or hate it, *Every Woman's Guide to Eating During Pregnancy* gives you all the practical information and tips you need to keep you and your baby healthy.

- *Nutrition for a Healthy Pregnancy: The Complete Guide to Eating Before, During, and After Your Pregnancy*
  Author: Elizabeth Somer; Publisher: Owl Books, September 2002
  An authoritative resource, this book includes the most current information linking maternal nutrition to infant behavior, birth defects, and other topics of concern, such as the physiological and emotional changes that occur during pregnancy.

- *Vegetarian Pregnancy: The Definitive Nutritional Guide to Having a Healthy Baby*
  Author: Sharon K Yntema; Publisher: Fireside Press, July 1993
  A sensible guide for women who want to enjoy a healthy pregnancy on a vegetarian diet. This book provides a complete, up-to-date resource to support the pregnant woman who chooses to be a vegetarian.

- *What to Eat When You're Expecting*
  Authors: Arlene Eisenberg, Heidi Murkoff, and Sandee Hathaway; Publisher: Workman Publishing Company, January 1986
  You are what you eat, and your baby is, too. Here is an easy-to-follow, up-to-date diet plan that uses a simple system to monitor servings from twelve food groups that promote fetal development and maternal well-being. The book offers 100 delicious recipes for nutritionally balanced meals, with special advice for vegetarians.

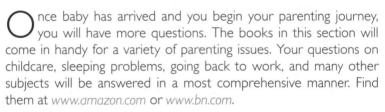

Chapter 27
Parenting Library

Once baby has arrived and you begin your parenting journey, you will have more questions. The books in this section will come in handy for a variety of parenting issues. Your questions on childcare, sleeping problems, going back to work, and many other subjects will be answered in a most comprehensive manner. Find them at *www.amazon.com* or *www.bn.com*.

○ Basic Childcare

Life with a newborn is exhilarating, exhausting, and at times it can be complicated. Babies don't come with instructions. Expectant parents are filled with anxieties, concerns, and questions about how to take care of and raise their new baby. Good basic childcare books can calm those anxieties, relieve concerns, and answer questions.

● *Baby Bargains*
Authors: Denise Fields and Alan Fields; Publisher: Windsor Peak Press, April 2005
Baby Bargains shows parents how to save money while selecting the best brands and the safest products for their baby.

● *Caring for Your Baby and Young Child: Birth to Age 5*
Author: American Academy of Pediatrics; Publisher: Bantam Books, June 2004
This book provides advice from the nation's leading specialists in pediatric medicine. It is especially helpful in explaining common health issues and immediately relieving worried parents about the many fears that often come with parenting a baby and young child.

● *On Becoming Babywise: The Classic Sleep Reference Guide*
Authors: Gary Ezzo and Robert Bucknam; Publisher: Parent-Wise Solutions, November 2001

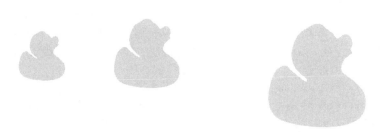

On Becoming Babywise brings hope to tired and bewildered parents looking for an alternative to sleepless nights and fussy babies. It teaches parents how to lovingly guide their baby's day, rather than being guided or enslaved by an infant's unknown needs.

- *Secrets of the Baby Whisperer: How to Calm, Connect, and Communicate with Your Baby*
  Authors: *Tracy Hogg and Melinda Blau*; Publisher: *Ballantine Books, January 2002*
  The key to a happy baby is understanding what she is trying to tell you with her cries, gestures, and facial expressions. In this book, Tracy Hogg unlocks the secrets of infant language so that any parent, grandparent, or caregiver can interpret what a baby is "saying" and give her what she needs. *Secrets of the Baby Whisperer* promises parents not only a healthier, happier baby, but a more relaxed and happy household.

- *The Girlfriends' Guide to Surviving the First Year of Motherhood*
  Author: *Vicki Lovine*; Publisher: *Perigee Trade, October 1997*
  The Girlfriends' Guide to Surviving the First Year of Motherhood is a first-time mother's must-have book. This is not a book about baby care; it's about caring for the new mom and the new family. Chapters on whether to work or not and resuming sexual activity are discussed with humor and honesty. Lovine will guide you through the dramatic emotions you experience as you transform from pregnant woman to mother.

- *The Happiest Baby on the Block: The New Way to Calm Crying and Help Your Newborn Baby Sleep Longer*
  Author: *Harvey Karp, M.D.*; Publisher: *Bantam Books, May 2003*

Dr. Karp believes that every baby is born with a "calming reflex," and that the secret to triggering it is replicating the conditions inside the womb. He recommends a series of five steps, which include swaddling, side/stomach position, shhh sounds, swinging, and sucking to calm your fussy baby. Parents who are at their wits' end because of a baby's incessant crying will find this book invaluable. Expectant parents may want to read it before they bring their newborn home from the hospital.

- *The Mother of All Baby Books: The Ultimate Guide to Your Baby's First Year*
  Author: Ann Douglas; Publisher: John Wiley & Sons, June 2002
  Covering everything imaginable, from newborn care and bathing basics to babyproofing your home and coping with sleepless nights, this valuable resource gives you lots of ways to nurture the new person in your life while still keeping your sanity. The author's well researched information and real-life tips will help you make this time more magical and memorable.

- *The Premature Baby Book: Everything You Need to Know About Your Premature Baby from Birth to Age One*
  Authors: William Sears, Robert Sears, James Sears, and Martha Sears; Publisher: Little, Brown & Company, September 2004
  If your baby is born prematurely, it's natural to be concerned. *The Premature Baby Book* offers the tools and advice you need to become comfortable with your potentially bewildering new role. Dr. Sears shows you how to become a valuable part of the medical team, helping your baby thrive by offering the care that only a parent can give.

- *What to Expect the First Year*
  Authors: Arlene Eisenberg, Heidi Murkoff, and Sandee Hathaway; Publisher: Workman Publishing, October 2003
  This comprehensive month-by-month guide clearly explains everything parents need to know about the first year with a new baby. Subjects include information on baby's monthly growth and development, feeding, sleeping habits, infant illnesses, safety, and much more.

○ Childcare for Multiples
Having multiples is a wonderful experience that can be exciting, fun, and easy if you get off to the right start. Keeping a schedule and following a routine make life much easier and happier for both you and the babies. Parents of multiples need more facts, more advice, more patience, and more support than most parents of singles. The following books will give you some ideas and suggestions about how to manage your life with multiples.

- *Mothering Multiples: Breastfeeding & Caring for Twins or More*
  Author: Karen Kerkhoff Gromada; Publisher: La Leche League International, July 1999

With an emphasis on attachment-style parenting, Gromada discusses parenting multiples from pregnancy and birth to toddlerhood, including infant care, maternal care, and more.

Buy "Mothering Multiples" today if you're serious about breastfeeding. This book has excellent information on breastfeeding your multiples.—Valerie

- *Raising Multiple Birth Children: A Parent's Survival Guide*
  Authors: *William and Sheila Laut*; Publisher: *Chandler House Press, June 1999*
  This book deals with the day-to-day adventures of parenting multiples. This is a must-have handbook for parents raising twins, triplets, quadruplets, and more; it's packed with practical tips and real-life solutions from multiple-birth parents.

- *The Art of Parenting Twins: The Unique Joys and Challenges of Raising Twins and Other Multiples*
  Authors: *Patricia Maxwell Malmstrom and Janet Poland*; Publisher: *Ballantine Publishing Group, June 1999*
  This complete, up-to-date guide will give you the skills you need to raise multiple-birth babies. Sections in this book include bonding with more than one baby, breastfeeding techniques, managing sibling rivalry, helping your children achieve independent identities, and more.

- *The Joy of Twins and Other Multiple Births: Raising and Loving Babies Who Arrive in Groups*
  Author: *Pamela Patrick Novotny*; Publisher: *Three Rivers Press, June 1994*
  A wonderful text that prepares you for postpregnancy, this book is scattered with beautiful photographs and focuses on the emotional health of new mothers, the babies, and the rest of the family.

- *The Multiples Manual: Preparing and Caring for Twins or Triplets*
  Author: *Lynn Lorenz*; Publisher: *Justmultiples.com, December 2003*
  This manual is guaranteed to simplify your life, save you time, and even save you money. A practical resource written with the expectant mother of multiples in mind.

- *Twins, Triplets, and More*
  Author: *Elizabeth M. Bryan*; Publisher: *St. Martin's Press, Inc., October 1998*
  This indispensable guide to multiple-birth parenting provides sensitive and practical solutions to twin- and triplet-related issues.

○ Same-Sex Couple Parenting

● *The Complete Lesbian and Gay Parenting Guide*
Author: Arlene Istar Lev; Publisher: Penguin, November 2004
This book covers every aspect of raising children in an alternative family setting. From issues that young children with same-sex parents may face in school to finding time for intimacy, it is a must have for LGTB couples who are thinking of raising children.

● *Gay Parenting: Complete Guide for Same-Sex Families*
Authors: Shana Priwer and Cynthia Phillips; Publisher: New Horizon Press, February 2006
This guide helps same-sex couples who are thinking of taking the next step to parenthood. It covers issues such as deciding whether to adopt, foster, or choose surrogacy, and how to accent family pride.

○ Preparing Your Own Baby Food
Although helping your baby establish healthy eating habits is not hard to do, starting solid foods can be an adventure. When your baby is ready to start eating solid foods, you'll want to prepare healthy, all-natural, age-appropriate meals using fresh, nutritious ingredients with no additives. This will help you make sure that your growing baby gets a balanced diet and establishes healthy eating habits from his toddler years through his adult life.

● *Baby Let's Eat*
Author: Rena Coyle; Publisher: Workman Publishing Company, November 1987
This kitchen-friendly cookbook offers great ideas for healthful meals and quick snacks without sugar or salt, and includes nutritional guidelines for children ages six months to three years.

● *First Meals*
Author: Annabel Karmel; Publisher: DK Publishing, Inc., May 2004
This book offers easy-to-follow, innovative recipes from baby's first solid foods to meals the whole family can enjoy. Nutritional information is provided for each recipe, as well as cooking times, freezing instructions, and suggestions for finicky or allergy-affected eaters.

● *Mommy Made and Daddy Too! Home Cooking for a Healthy Baby and Toddler*
Authors: Martha Kimmel, David Kimmel, and Suzanne Goldenson; Publisher: Bantam Books, June 2000
Mommy Made and Daddy Too! is filled with 140 easy-to-make recipes that are prefect for introducing your baby to wholesome solid foods. These delicious, kid-tested dishes—which include finger foods, shakes and smoothies, snacks on the go, and a variety of table dishes—were created with your baby's special nutritional needs in mind, and they will help your child establish healthy eating habits that will last a lifetime.

- *Super Baby Food*
  Author: Ruth Yaron; Publisher: F J Roberts Publishing Company, June 1998
  Learn everything about feeding your baby and toddler solid foods during her first three years. This book will tell you how and when to start your baby on solid foods, with detailed information on the best and safest highchairs, spoons, bibs, and other feeding equipment.

○ Mother and Baby Workout Books
  Working out with your baby is a wonderful way to have fun and spend quality time together while you get back into shape. Babies will love being lifted, rolled around, and simply being held close. These books will get you started.

- *Baby Om: Yoga for Mothers and Babies*
  Authors: Laura Staton and Sarah Perron; Publisher: Owl Books, August 2002
  Baby Om takes mothers through a yoga practice they can do with their infants any time, anywhere. The techniques help new mothers enjoy the spiritual and physical benefits of yoga and allow them to nurture themselves, as well as their babies.

- *Bounce Back Into Shape After Baby: The Ultimate Guide to a Fun-Filled, Time- and Energy-Efficient Workout with Your Baby*
  Author: Caroline Corning Creager; Publisher: Executive Physical Therapy, September 2002
  New mothers will benefit from these postpartum exercise ideas. Photos depicting full-body stretching and strengthening workouts are complemented by helpful advice on tightening abdominal muscles, exercising with baby, improving posture, and more.

- *Yoga Mom, Buddha Baby: The Yoga Workout for New Moms*
  Author: Jyothi Larson; Publisher: Bantam Books, April 2002
  Practicing yoga with your baby as you hold her, have her next to you, or have her leaning against your thighs or atop your belly is a wonderful way to add to your first year together.

This is a book that has simple exercises done with your baby and illustrated with clear and beautiful photos of moms actually doing this!—Connie

○ Avoiding and Correcting Sleeping Problems
  If your child isn't sleeping, chances are you're not sleeping either, and a good night's sleep is crucial both for a child's well-being and a parent's peace of mind. These books help parents establish good sleeping habits for their children. They offer tips and techniques on how to handle the problems that cause sleepless nights, from colic to bedwetting to nightmares. Learn how to

make bedtime and naptime stress free for yourself and your child. Establishing good sleep habits right from the beginning can prevent a lot of problems down the road. Some of the issues addressed in these books are:

✔ The common mistakes parents make to get their children to sleep, including the inclination to rock and feed.
✔ Exploring the different sleep cycle needs for different temperaments, from quiet babies to hyperactive toddlers.
✔ How long you should let your baby cry before sleep.
✔ When to start scheduling naps.
✔ Whether you should wake baby for a feeding.
✔ How routines affect your child's sleep.
✔ What sleep patterns are normal for babies and children.
✔ How to prevent a two-year-old from having a tantrum at the words "Time for bed."
✔ How to help your child cope with nighttime fears.

- *Healthy Sleep Habits, Happy Child*
  Author: Marc Weissbluth; Publisher: Ballantine Publishing, April 1999
  This book addresses your children's sleep habits as they move from infancy into adolescence. Dr. Marc Weissbluth explains with authority and reassurance his step-by-step regimen for instituting beneficial habits within the framework of your child's natural sleep cycles.

- *Sleeping Through the Night*
  Author: Jodi A Mindell; Publisher: HarperCollins, March 2005
  A child psychologist presents what all new parents so desperately need—a simple and accessible guide to getting babies and toddlers to fall asleep and stay asleep.

- *Solve Your Child's Sleep Problems*
  Author: Richard Ferber; Publisher: Simon & Schuster, April 1986
  The director of the Sleep Laboratory and Center for Pediatric Sleep Disorders at Children's Hospital in Boston provides safe, sound ideas for helping a child fall asleep and stay asleep. New parents will benefit from Ferber's advice on developing good sleeping patterns and daily schedules to ensure that sleeping problems don't develop in the first place.

- *The No-Cry Sleep Solution*
  Author: Elizabeth Pantley; Publisher: McGraw-Hill, March 2002
  This book offers gentle ways to help your baby sleep through the night. Elizabeth Pantley's guide provides you with effective strategies for overcoming naptime and nighttime problems. *The No-Cry Sleep*

Solution offers clearly explained, step-by-step ideas that steer your little ones toward a good night's sleep with no crying.

○ Single Mothering
Being a single parent isn't easy. Whether you're a single mom by choice or chance, these books provide you with the understanding, support, and knowledge you'll need to be a good single parent. They talk about key issues such as getting organized, managing the household, balancing family and work, creating a financial plan, dealing with difficult emotions, finding high-quality child care, creating a support network, and much more.

● *Complete Single Mother: Reassuring Answers to Your Most Challenging Concerns*
  Authors: Andrea Engber and Leah Klungness; Publisher: Adams Media Corp, March 2006
  Filled with expert information and pragmatic advice, this comprehensive and practical reference answers questions concerning resolving custody issues, managing your finances, dealing with an irresponsible ex, handling work pressures, collecting child support, and many more.

● *Single Mothers by Choice: A Guidebook for Single Women Who Are Considering or Have Chosen Motherhood*
  Author: Jane Mattes; Publisher: Three Rivers Press, May 1994
  This is the first handbook for the rapidly growing number of American women who choose single motherhood. Mattes presents an accessible and personal analysis of the available options, and examines the problems, questions, and rewards of single motherhood.

● *The Single Mom's Workplace Survival Guide: A Practical Guide*
  Author: Brenda Armstrong; Publisher: Servant Publications, August 2002
  In this practical and encouraging book, single parent and financial counselor Brenda Armstrong shows single mothers how to meet the challenges of the workplace, avoid mistakes, prepare for the effort, develop a plan for the future, and survive with success.

● *The Single Mother's Survival Guide*
  Author: Patrice Karst; Publisher: Crossing Press, Inc., March 2000
  Patrice Karst, a single mother, shares her practical and witty advice with single moms everywhere. She covers a wide range of topics that relate to the modern woman struggling without a mate, showing how it's possible not only to survive, but to triumph.

Whenever I'm feeling overwhelmed about the situation I'm in, I pick up this book and regain my center, my focus, and my goals for life.—Donna

○ Mothers Going Back to Work

If they have to or want to go back to work, many women develop guilt feelings about leaving their children. However, research shows that a satisfied working mother may influence her children more positively and provide a better role model than an unhappy stay-at-home mom. Whether single or married, with one child or more, every working mother must find her own way of balancing home and work. Is the priority career or motherhood? Do you have to sacrifice one to be successful in the other? Is it really possible to have it all? These books will help to answer some of the questions often asked by working mothers.

- *Getting It Right: How Working Mothers Successfully Take Up the Challenge of Life, Family, and Career*
  Author: Laraine T. Zappert; Publisher: Simon & Schuster, March 2002
  Laraine Zappert guides parents through decisions about such crucial issues as timing the birth of their children, allocating housework, evaluating various work arrangements, and lining up support. Though there is much to be gained from them, her time-tested solutions for creating a healthy balance between work and home require effort and dedication.

- *When Mothers Work: Loving Our Children Without Sacrificing Ourselves*
  Author: Joan K. Peters; Publisher: Perseus Books, September 1998
  Most mothers today face the challenge of balancing work and family, and they often feel it's a struggle to manage both roles well. This book takes on the myth of the perfect mother and the pressure on women from society to embody that role.

- *Working Mothers 101*
  Author: Katherine Wyse Goldman; Publisher: HarperCollins, June 1998
  In this book, you'll find practical strategies for working mothers who are trying to make their lives and homes run smoothly. Here's everything you need to know when you want to get control of your time, your life, and your future.

○ Discipline

We all want to raise happy, well-adjusted, well-behaved children, and we all have to use discipline at one time or another to do that. But many parents are unsure of exactly how to discipline their children and what methods to use. The following books answer those questions and contain helpful tools parents can use to create family harmony and improve family communication.

- *The Discipline Book: How to Have a Better-Behaved Child from Birth to Age Ten*
  Authors: Martha Sears and William Sears; Publisher: Little Brown & Company, February 1995
  This book focuses on preventing behavior problems before they start and managing them when they arise. Topics discussed are self-esteem,

spanking, divorce, single parenting, travel, and babysitting, as well as other disciplinary issues and practices.

- *The Fussy Baby Book: Parenting Your High-Need Child from Birth to Age Five*
  Author: William Sears; Publisher: Little, Brown and Company, September 1996
  If your child is a real handful, parenting can be exhausting and frustrating. This reassuring book explains how to recognize whether your child is high-need and how to best respond and relate to her if she is.

○ Welcoming a Second Child
Many parents are surprised at how different the situation feels when the second child arrives. Even before the birth, there are all kinds of questions such as: "Can we possibly love a second child as much as the first? Is it better to have them close in age or further apart? What about sibling rivalry?" The books described here will help answer these and other questions you'll have when you're expecting, and after you deliver, your second child.

- *And Baby Makes Four: Welcoming a Second Child into the Family*
  Author: Hilory Wagner; Publisher: HarperCollins, August 1998
  And Baby Makes Four is written to inform and support each member of the family as they meet the challenges that come with welcoming another child. Hilory Wagner provides a one-of-a kind reference to guide parents through the many changes that affect their growing family.

- *From One Child to Two: What to Expect, How to Cope, and How to Enjoy Your Growing Family*
  Author: Judy Dunn; Publisher: Ballantine Books, January 1995
  Judy Dunn gives parents all the information, emotional support, and reassurance they need to minimize the conflicts and relish the joys of raising two children.

- *The New Baby at Your House*
  Authors: Joanna Cole and Margaret Miller; Publisher: HarperTrophy, March 1999
  Written for young children, this reassuring book prepares them for the ups and downs of having a new baby in the house.

- *Twice Blessed*
  Author: Joan Leonard; Publisher: St. Martin's Press, March 2000
  Second-time parenting brings its own set of questions, quandaries, and chaos, and *Twice Blessed* helps you prepare for the changes that are about to occur. Issues covered include preparing for a different pregnancy and birth, preparing for another dramatic change in your marriage, and preparing your child for a new brother or sister.

- *Welcoming Your Second Baby*
  Author: Vicki Lansky; Publisher: Book Peddlers, July 2005
  Vicki Lansky has compiled a book of suggestions to help make the transition from only child to big brother or sister a smooth one. She

presents helpful tips, including how to address feelings of jealousy, how to help your child cope while you're away in the hospital, and how to include your first child in this remarkable event.

Vicki Lansky answers all of your questions about being pregnant with another baby! Everything from how to handle your toddler while pregnant to bringing that baby home!—Sandy

○ Siblings Welcoming a New Baby
Bringing a new baby home can sometimes be a traumatic event for an older sibling. A new baby can cause changes and disruptions in the life of the older child. Your firstborn child may welcome a new brother or sister with mixed emotions. Feelings of love and tenderness may be present one minute, anger and jealousy the next. Although it's an exciting time for the older child, now there's someone else in the family demanding Mom and Dad's love and attention. The books that follow are all written for young children, and they will help answer your child's questions about what new babies look like, what they do and don't do, and what it will really be like to have one around the house.

● *I'm a Big Brother* or *I'm a Big Sister*
Author: Joanna Cole; Publisher: HarperCollins, April 1997
These two books are written specifically either for girls or for boys, depending on the gender of the older sibling. If your older child is a girl, the word sister will mean so much to her in defining her identity after a baby joins the family, and the same thing applies to big brothers. Each simple, first-person text tells what babies like, why they cry, what they're too little to do, and how much parents love their older children.

● *Our New Baby*
Author: Wendy Cheyette Lewison; Publisher: Grosset and Dunlap, October 1996
Having a new baby is fun, but it also takes some getting used to. This appealing, photo-filled book reassures siblings that they are still very special to their parents and proves that a little newcomer can be nice to have around.

● *We Have a Baby*
Author: Cathryn Falwell; Publisher: Clarion Books, March 1999
This is the perfect book for a new or about-to-be big sister or big brother. It introduces the important things the whole family can do for the baby and shows all the love the baby will give in return.

- *What to Expect When Mommy's Having a Baby*
  Author: Heidi E. Murkoff; Publisher: HarperCollins, January 2004
  With the help of Angus, the lovable "Answer Dog," children are provided with answers to many of the questions they may have about their mother's pregnancy. Some of the issues the book addresses are how the baby grows, where the baby is, how long it will be there, why Mommy is sick sometimes, and how the baby comes out to join the family.

- *What to Expect When the New Baby Comes Home*
  Author: Heidi E. Murkoff; Publisher: HarperCollins, December 2000
  After months of preparation, anticipation, and a bit of anxiety, the new baby is coming home. Angus, the lovable "Answer Dog," helps toddlers and preschoolers make the transition from only child to older sibling. This book addresses basic questions such as "What do new babies eat?" and "Why do new babies cry so much?" to more significant concerns like "Why do new babies get so many presents?"

○ Sibling Rivalry
Sibling rivalry is inevitable. Siblings often feel jealous, resentful, or in competition with one another. These books offer solutions to constant squabbling and emotional upsets. They teach parents how to stop encouraging competition between children by acknowledging individual talents and skills without comparison. In the books that follow, parents will find practical guidelines and tools for reducing friction among children and resolving sibling conflicts.

- *Beyond Sibling Rivalry: How to Help Your Children Become Cooperative, Caring, and Compassionate*
  Author: Peter Goldenthal; Publisher: Owl Books, February 2000
  This book talks about children's relationships in the context of the family as a whole. It provides practical guidelines and tools for reducing friction among children, and explains how to recognize and highlight each child's unique abilities and interests.

- *Birth Order Blues*
  Author: Meri Wallace; Publisher: Owl Books, May 1999
  The author raises parents' awareness of the impact of birth order on children and suggests ways to resolve or circumvent potential problems. Learn to identify specific birth-order problems such as underachievement and aggression, among many others. Also, learn how to replace negative behavior problems with positive reinforcement and habits.

- *Siblings Without Rivalry: How to Help Your Children Live Together So You Can Live, Too*
  Authors: Adele Faber and Elaine Mazlish; Publisher: HarperCollins, December 2004
  If you have more than one child, you'll find this book invaluable. It offers helpful information you can use to teach your children to get along, and

help them overcome the fear that one might not get his share of love and attention from you, or that a sibling will accomplish more. It teaches you how to understand and cope with your children's resentment of one another, and how to encourage good feelings within the family.

If you have more than one child and want to understand the rivalry and bickering and learn ways to improve your children's relationship with each other, then read this book.—Jill

- The Baffled Parent's Guide to Sibling Rivalry
  Author: Marian Edelman Borden; Publisher: McGraw-Hill, May 2003
  This resource provides parents with advice on how to keep relative peace in the family. Organized for easy access by topics that provoke the largest number of arguments among siblings (such as room sharing and borrowing toys, as well as issues related to step- and half-siblings), these effective solutions help parents sort through how and when to intervene.

○ Medical Advice and Emergency and First-Aid Treatment
  If your child is sick or there's an emergency, always call your doctor first. For answers to questions about common and not-so-common ailments and emergencies, refer to one of these books for medical advice and emergency and first-aid treatment.

  - American Medical Association Complete Guide to Your Children's Health
    Author: American Medical Association; Publisher: Random House, December 1998
    Part 1 of the *American Medical Association Complete Guide to Your Children's Health* covers birth through adolescence, with chapters on everything from feeding and bathing newborns to answering difficult questions about sexuality. Part 2 deals with making the right choices for your child's well-being, including finding the best day care and how to pick a pediatrician. Part 3 is a comprehensive medical encyclopedia, with detailed information on more than 300 childhood maladies.

  - Baby and Child Emergency First-Aid Handbook: Simple Step-by-Step Instructions for the Most Common Childhood Emergencies
    Author: Mitchell J. Einzig; Publisher: Meadowbrook, November 1992
    When an emergency occurs, don't panic. Pick up this user-friendly book. Designed to provide parents with clear, concise, easy-to-follow directions in seconds, this handbook offers step-by-step, illustrated instructions for thirty-four of the most common childhood emergencies.

- *The Children's Hospital Guide to Your Child's Health and Development*
  Author: Children's Hospital Boston; Publisher: Perseus Publishing, November 2002
  This book offers all the medical, psychological, and practical information you need to raise healthy children from birth through elementary school. It's packed full of information on symptoms, causes, diagnosis, treatment, and prevention of common medical problems, and it includes vital, up-to-date advice for choosing medical care and insurance, and for finding good childcare. *The Children's Hospital Guide* includes charts of normal development at all ages and a comprehensive resource section.

- *The American Academy of Pediatrics Guide to Your Child's Symptoms: The Official, Complete Home Reference, Birth Through Adolescence*
  Authors: Donald Schiff and Steven Shelov; Publisher: Random House, September 1997
  An A-to-Z directory of more than 100 of the most common childhood symptoms, presented in clearly illustrated, easy-to-follow charts designed to enable a parent to quickly identify a symptom, learn its possible cause, and determine how best to proceed, whether it's taking action at home or calling the pediatrician.

○ Child Safety
Safety is the first concern in the minds of new parents. Making your house, garage, and backyard safe is one of the most important things you'll ever do for your child. Start early. It is essential for your child's well-being. The books listed here provide excellent guidelines for keeping your child safe.

- *Baby Proofing Basics*
  Author: Vicki Lansky; Publisher: Book Peddlers, September 2002
  Baby Proofing Basics is a detailed and practical guide for babyproofing your home. The book reviews commonly available child-safety products and talks about safety strategies for your home, as well as when you're out visiting others. It also includes sections on holiday safety, outdoor play safety, and poison prevention and action. There are guidelines and checklists for child proofing your child's environment room by room and situation by situation. This book is a well-thought-out guide to keeping toddlers and young children safe and healthy.

- *Child Safe: A Practical Guide for Preventing Childhood Injuries*
  Author: Mark A. Brandenberg; Publisher: Three Rivers Press, March 2000
  Child Safe is a valuable guide to identifying the potential hazards a child can encounter at home and school, on the playground, and in the car.

- *Child Safety Made Easy*
  Authors: Lori Marques and Lisa Carter; Publisher: Screamin' Mimi Publications, December 1998

Eliminate the dangers surrounding your children by learning how to childproof your home. Brief and to the point, this book is full of good advice that can greatly reduce the incidence of accidents in your home and outdoors.

○ Traveling with Small Children

Traveling with small children can be a chore. When busy moms and dads go on vacation, the last thing they need is to deal with kid-related catastrophes, fits, and disasters. Traveling with children may sound like a recipe for disaster, but with the right information and advice, traveling with your children can be a wonderful, stress-free experience.

Every family is different and has its own sense of adventure, budget issues, and stresses. When you are planning a family vacation, look at all of your options, and consider your family's likes and dislikes. Figure out, as a family, what you enjoy, what you don't like, and what sort of shared experience would work best, and then plan accordingly. If you take the time to plan and do the research, you can save time and money, and have the kind of vacation you and your family can afford and enjoy. These books offer ideas, tips, and suggestions for making traveling with small children easy and fun.

● *Fodor's FYI: Travel with Your Baby: Experts Share Their Secrets*
Author: Fodor's; Publisher: Fodor's, June 2001

Fodor's globe-trotting parents show you how you can take your kids just about anywhere. Get great advice on zeroing in on the best-bet vacations for newborns, toddlers, and preschoolers, as well as traveling smart to the beach, the city, and the countryside, here and abroad. Tried-and-true strategies for getting the best deals wherever you go, finding the most family-friendly hotels, packing, childproofing your hotel room, eating smart, and other secrets of whine-free vacationing.

● *On the Go with Baby: A Stress-Free Guide to Getting Across Town or Around the World*
Author: Ericka Lutz; Publisher: Sourcebooks, April 2002

If you have young children and enjoy stepping beyond your front porch, *On the Go with Baby* is your resource for practical advice on packing, choosing a vacation, babyproofing a hotel room, handling public tantrums, and dealing with anything else that could possibly happen outside the home. Ericka Lutz will show you the basics of boldly going anywhere.

○ Baby Record Books

The first year of a child's life is a magical time of growth and discovery. At no other time are physical changes and developmental achievements so dramatic. Keeping a baby record book lets you record all the wonderful events, special milestones, and accomplishments of your baby and relive them with your child in the decades ahead.

- *Baby's First Year Journal*
  Author: A. Christine Harris; Publisher: Chronicle Books, July 1999
  Baby's First Year Journal is the perfect place for parents to record their little one's accomplishments and their own observations while they learn about baby's early social, physical, and cognitive development.

- *Baby Memory Books*
  Publisher: C. R. Gibson
  Web sites: *www.crgibson.com*; *www.babycatalog.com*; *www.kidsurplus.com*
  Classic C. R. Gibson memory books have been a favorite for generations. These books include space for you to record all the important events that take place during baby's first year.

- *My First Five Years: A Record of Early Childhood*
  Author : Anne Geddes; Publisher: Andrews McMeel Publishing, April 2005
  Web sites: *www.amazon.com*; *www.annegeddes.com*; *www.bn.com*
  Babies grow and change each day, and every moment is an opportunity for discovery. This exceptional book helps parents record the milestones, memories, firsts, and favorites as their infant becomes a toddler and their toddler heads off to school.

○ Memory Books for Twins
Multiples are special, each in his or her own way. They each have different personalities, likes, and dislikes. Because they are individuals, it's nice to keep separate memory books. The books that follow will help you do that.

- *Double Time: A Helpful Book of Schedule Keeping for Twins*
  Publisher: Double Blessings
  Web site: *www.doubleblessings.com*. Search under "calendars."
  Keep track of feedings, diapering, medications, naps, and other important information with these easy-to-use, daily schedules designed just for twins!

- *The Story of Me Baby Memory Book—Twins Combo*
  Publisher: n/a
  Web site: *www.baby-memory-books.com*
  The Story of Me twins combo is a perfect choice for new baby twins. The combo includes two complete baby memory books, along with two sets of "More than Me" page packs, with modified pages designed to fit the needs of families with twins.

- Twin Dreaming of Hunny (set of two bound baby memory books)
  Publisher: C. R. Gibson
  Web sites: *www.kidsurplus.com*; *www.mymamabear.com*
  These adorable "We Are Twins" memory books feature classic "Dreaming of Hunny" Winnie the Pooh artwork. These colorful albums include decorative pages designed to record all of your twins' first milestones through the first five years.

Chapter 28

Video and DVD Library

In addition to reading up on what to expect and how to stay fit, expectant and new parents might find videos an indispensable resource on a wide range of topics. If you prefer visual aids, or you just want to sit back and relax while you learn, these videos are a great choice.

○ Pregnancy and Childbirth

Sit and relax with your husband or birth partner and enjoy these instructional videos in the privacy of your own home. Learn about conception, labor, delivery, and birth. Keep fit during and after pregnancy with prenatal exercise videos. Learn how to relax and enjoy a stress-free pregnancy by practicing yoga. These videos will answer many of your questions and prepare you for this wonderful experience.

• Baby Time: Baby to Be—The Video Guide to Pregnancy
Studio: View Inc.
VHS/DVD Release Date, April 2002
Web sites: *www.amazon.com*; *www.bn.com*
This video is designed to help expectant parents through some of the difficult times they may face as they prepare for parenthood. Maryjane Henning focuses on prenatal care, nutrition, embryonic development, changes to Mom's body and mood, and how all of these matters affect Dad.

• Childbirth from Inside Out, Part I: Pregnancy and the Prenatal Period
Studio: View, Inc.
VHS/DVD Release Date, July 2003
Web sites: *www.amazon.com*; *www.bn.com*

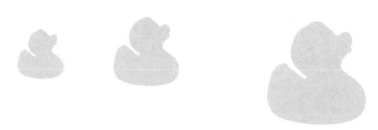

This film is the first part of a two-part program that informs parents-to-be on the fundamentals of childbirth. Part I addresses the period of time from conception through gestation. The miraculous development of the embryo is traced and the profound impact of pregnancy on the mother's body is presented.

- Childbirth from Inside Out, Part 2: Delivery and the Postnatal Period
  Studio: View, Inc.
  VHS/DVD Release Date, September 2003
  Web sites: *www.amazon.com*; *www.bn.com*
  Part 2 of this video starts with the miracle of the birthing experience and goes through some principles of postnatal care. The film is designed to familiarize the expectant couple with the beginning of labor; it then follows the childbirth process from checking in at the hospital through the delivery.

- Expecting Multiples
  Studio: Multiple Birth Resources LLC
  VHS Release Date, December 1999
  Web site: *www.expectingmultiples.com*
  Multiple Birth Resources LLC specializes in educating and preparing expectant parents for pregnancy, delivery, and life with more than one baby. This comprehensive 151-minute double video series will show you how to be proactive with your multiple pregnancy and decrease the chances of premature delivery and low-birth-weight babies.

- Having Your Baby: A Complete Lamaze Prepared Childbirth Class
  Studio: Pearent Productions
  VHS/DVD Release Date, June 2004
  Web sites: *www.amazon.com*; *www.bn.com*; *www.fitbeginnings.com*
  If you can't attend a childbirth class, this video will bring the class to you. *Having Your Baby* is the only complete step-by-step instructional video on Lamaze-prepared childbirth available today. Lamaze seeks to reduce pain through relaxation achieved by massage, focus, and a series of breathing techniques.

I really wanted to be able to learn about Lamaze and childbirth techniques in the privacy of my own home. I purchased this hoping to get the basics down and this DVD provided that and more.—Kirsten

- Labor of Love Childbirth Class
  Studio: Repnet
  VHS/DVD Release Date, February 2004
  Web sites: *www.amazon.com*; *www.bn.com*; *www.childbirthclass.com*
  In this program, which is meant to be watched over two days, Sherry Turney addresses third-trimester experiences, breathing techniques, stages of labor, comfort suggestions, epidurals, birth positions, and possible medical interventions.

○ Prenatal Exercise
  Exercising during pregnancy will improve your overall energy level and stamina, relieve discomfort, and improve posture, circulation, and digestion. Before you start any exercise program, be sure to check with your doctor.

- Denise Austin Mat Workout Based on the Work of J. H. Pilates
  Studio: Lions Gate
  VHS/DVD Release Date, March 2001
  Web sites: *www.amazon.com*; *www.bn.com*
  Denise Austin's Mat Workout presents two 20-minute workouts that emphasize flexibility, core strength, and relaxation. Workout 1 is Pilates based and focuses on the core muscles of the abdominal area and back. Workout 2 includes yoga poses that emphasize balance and flexibility, and Pilates-based exercises that focus on core stability and strength.

- Denise Austin Pregnancy Plus Workout
  Studio: Artisan Entertainment
  VHS Release Date, November 1998

Web site: *www.amazon.com*

This video features a total fitness program that will keep you in shape both before and after your baby is born. Famous for her cheerleading style, Denise Austin packs this program with energetic aerobics, helpful posture and breathing tips, substantial advice, and plenty of TLC.

- Kathy Smith Pregnancy Workout
  Studio: Sony Wonder
  VHS/DVD Release Date, March 2002
  Web site: *www.amazon.com*; *www.bn.com*; *www.fitnessbeginnings.com*
  This workout video helps expectant moms prepare their bodies for labor and delivery, and get back into shape after giving birth. Both prenatal and postnatal segments include warm-ups, stretches, aerobic routines, and toning exercises for the entire body.

- Leisa Hart's FitMama: Prenatal Workout
  Studio: Goldhil Home Media
  VHS/DVD Release Date, April 2003
  Web site: *www.fitnessbeginnings.com*
  This workout program is broken into four different segments: "Salsa Dance" introduces easy-to-follow, low-impact moves; "Yoga Fat Burn" targets every major muscle group with emphasis on the hips and thighs; "Labor and Delivery Prep" helps build abdominal strength, combined with Kegel exercises to strengthen pelvic floor muscles; and "Prenatal Stretch and Relax" focuses on easing back discomfort with stretching as you concentrate on labor and delivery breathing techniques.

○ Prenatal Yoga
Yoga is a safe, relaxing way to exercise, and yoga workouts can be done through all stages of pregnancy. Yoga techniques focus on achieving benefits such as learning how to relax and relieving discomfort and stress. Yoga includes stretches and strength-building exercises, which help prepare the expectant mom for labor and birth.

- Crunch: Yoga Mama—Prenatal Yoga
  Studio: Anchor Bay
  VHS/DVD Release Date, April 2004
  Web sites: *www.amazon.com*; *www.bn.com*; *www.fitnessbeginnings.com*
  This video offers a safety-conscious, simple, straightforward workout with real potential for increased strength and flexibility. Intensive techniques focus on clearing the mind, keeping the body healthy, and connecting emotionally with your baby.

- Prenatal Yoga with Shiva Rea
  Studio: Living Arts
  VHS/DVD Release Date, February 2004
  Web sites: *www.amazon.com*; *www.fitnessbeginnings.com*

Shiva Rea presents a unique series of stretches and strength-building exercises for pregnant women. Exercises include modifications for each trimester. Ms. Rea has made a tape with the flexibility to carry an expectant mom throughout her entire pregnancy and beyond.

- Prenatal Yoga with Colette Crawford
  Studio: Injoy Studios
  VHS Release Date, April 1996
  Web site: *www.amazon.com*
  Certified Iyengar yoga instructor and registered nurse Colette Crawford guides viewers through a gentle routine designed to strengthen muscles, alleviate common prenatal discomforts (sciatica, back pain, leg cramps), and restore energy.

- The New Method—Baby & Mom Prenatal Yoga
  Studio: Parage
  VHS Release Date, July 2001
  Web sites: *www.bn.com*; *www.fitnessbeginnings.com*
  This video provides simple and effective exercises specifically geared to strengthen and relax your rapidly changing body. Gurmuka Kaur Khalsa discusses the role of yoga in helping with pregnancy.

○ Postnatal Exercises

Many women gain weight during pregnancy, and many find it difficult to get back to their old weight and shape after they give birth. Get back into shape the fun, easy way with these postnatal videos. Trim down and firm up after giving birth. Doing the exercises on these videos will help you lose pounds and inches, flatten your tummy, reclaim a trim waistline, and build up your energy.

- Denise Austin Bounce Back After Baby
  Studio: Artisan Entertainment
  VHS Release Date, August 2000
  Web site: *www.bn.com*
  Bounce Back After Baby is a workout video that offers a special exercise routine designed to help new mothers lose weight, firm up, and increase their energy. The video offers 20 minutes of low-impact, high-energy aerobic workouts. A 15-minute toning segment targets the abdominal area, hips, thighs, and buttocks with traditional floor-work exercises (no weights). The workout ends with a renewing, peaceful 10 minutes of stretch and relaxation, and a special bonus routine for women who have had a Cesarean section.

- Cindy Crawford A New Dimension
  Studio: Good Times Home Video
  VHS/DVD Release Date, April 2000
  Web sites: *www.amazon.com*; *www.bn.com*

This program includes two short, easy workouts, and one long one. Workout A (12 minutes) is a light-intensity routine with mostly stretching and some strength moves such as lunges and abdominal curls. Workout B (16 minutes) includes cardio moves that are simple and low-impact, such as knee lifts, marching, squats, lunges, crunches, and pushups. Workout C (41 minutes) is a full-body workout that consists mostly of muscle endurance, with some segments of cardiovascular exercise.

○ Mother and Baby Workouts

The responsibilities of caring for a newborn can be overwhelming, and the sleep-deprived new mother often puts her own physical condition low on the priority list. Exercising with these videos is the ideal way to get back into shape while you care for and play with your baby. There's no need to go to the gym or hire a babysitter. Now you can get back into shape while you spend quality time with your baby, all in the comfort and convenience of your own home.

● Complete Body Workout for Mom and Baby—Postnatal Fitness
Studio: Tapeworm
VHS Release Date, March 1999
Web site: *www.amazon.com*
Becky Cortez presents this 46-minute workout tape for new mothers, which includes a stretch warm-up, a 17-minute cardio workout, 12 minutes of toning and conditioning, an abs segment, and a cooldown stretch. The toning segment uses an exercise band and weights as well. Babies join their moms as Cortez explains how to do push-ups over the infants. Babies also join their moms during the cooldown segment and for the four-minute "baby play" at the end, which includes a little stretching and a little baby dancing.

○ Newborn Care

New parents often have a million questions and are sometimes embarrassed to ask many of them for fear of seeming unprepared for the task that lies ahead. These videos provide new parents with the answers to many of the questions and situations that arise when a new baby comes home from the hospital.

● Baby Time—Baby Talk: The Video Guide for New Parents
Studio: Peter Pan
VHS/DVD Release Date, April 2002
Web sites: *www.amazon.com*; *www.bn.com*
Endorsed by The American Academy of Pediatrics, this program details how to care for a newborn and provides answers to a number of questions that nearly every parent wonders about.

● Baby Time Series: First Days Home—Keeping Your Baby Healthy & Happy
Studio: Peter Pan

VHS/DVD Release Date, April 2002

Web site: *www.amazon.com*

New parents need all the help and advice they can get for taking care of their newborn baby during their first days at home. This informative video includes topics such as baby's appearance, breastfeeding, formula feeding, sleeping, crying and comforting, bathing, diapering and dressing, baby's health, safety, and more.

- The Happiest Baby on the Block
  Studio: Trinity Home Entertainment
  VHS/DVD Release Date, March 2003
  Web sites: *www.amazon.com*; *www.bn.com*; *www.colicshop.com*
  Pediatrician Harvey Karp has developed a baby-soothing system for fussy and colicky babies. Dr. Karp believes that every baby is born with a "calming reflex," and that the secret to triggering it is replicating the conditions inside the womb. He'll walk you through the five easy-to-follow techniques that his devoted followers absolutely swear by.

○ Baby Massage

Soothe and nurture your baby through massage. It's a great way to bond and spend quality time with your baby.

- Brighter Baby
  Studio: Wellspring Media
  VHS/DVD Release Date, November 2003
  Web sites: *www.amazon.com*; *www.bn.com*; *www.videouniverse.com*
  Brenda Adderly hosts this special program on the effects of baby care on brain development and intelligence. Ms. Adderly guides the viewer through examples and demonstrations of how one can influence a baby's mental development through certain types of activities, such as massages and the controversial Mozart theory.

- Gift of Baby Massage
  Studio: Consumervision Inc.
  VHS Release Date, January 2002
  Web sites: *www.amazon.com*; *www.bn.com*
  In this video, certified massage therapist Rebecca Klinger and pediatrician Max Kahn show you how to give your baby an infant massage. They also answer frequently asked questions on topics such as how often to massage, when to massage, and at what age to begin massaging your baby.

- Gentle Touch Infant Massage
  Studio: Goldhil Home Media
  VHS Release Date, October 2003
  Web sites: *www.amazon.com*; *www.gentletouchparent-child.com*

Gentle Touch Infant Massage is a step-by-step lesson in learning a practical and enjoyable massage technique for your infant.

○ Getting Your Baby to Sleep
Nearly half of all new parents struggle nightly with their baby's sleep problems. The resulting stress, sleep deprivation, and exhaustion are a chronic problem for millions of parents and children. These videos present a clear, simple, and effective method of getting your baby to sleep.

- It's Sleepy Time
  Studio: Video Distributors, Inc.
  VHS Release Date, September 1998
  Web site: *www.amazon.com*
  Created with the experts at Duke University Medical Center, this video demonstrates bedtime rituals for parents to follow when putting infants to sleep for the night. Guiding children through nighttime fears and showing parents how to handle problem sleepers is what this reassuring video is all about.

- Your Baby Can Sleep
  Studio: Better Health Video, Inc.
  DVD Release Date, July 2005
  Web site: *www.amazon.com*
  With the help of Dr. Stewart Tomaras, a pediatric sleep specialist, you can have your baby sleeping well in about a week. Dr. Tomaras outlines five specific stages of achieving good sleep: creating good sleep associations, a bedtime routine, a transition period, crying, and "the plan." This is a wonderfully detailed plan for getting your baby to sleep well.

○ Classical Music for Babies
It's never too early to introduce your baby to the world of classical music. Listening to classical music has been shown to enhance creativity, improve academic achievement, reduce anxiety, and heighten mental awareness. Music therapy research has shown that listening to classical music can produce positive effects on health and well-being.

- Baby Bach Musical Adventure
  Studio: Buena Vista Entertainment
  VHS/DVD Release Date, March 2002
  Web sites: *www.amazon.com*; *www.babyeinstein.com*
  Captivating images accompany baby-friendly arrangements of Bach's music. Designed for infants and toddlers, "Baby Bach" features familiar toys and colorful objects moving to the beautiful music of Johann Sebastian Bach.

- Baby Beethoven Symphony of Fun
  Studio: Buena Vista Home Entertainment
  VHS/DVD Release Date, October 2002

Web sites: *www.amazon.com*; *www.babycenter.com*; *www.babyeinstein.com*
A series of engaging, baby-friendly images such as toys, puppets, and art are set to Beethoven's music that has been reorchestrated for children.

My son loves the bright colors, moving objects, toys, animals, and music.—Jennifer

- Baby Mozart Music Festival
  Studio: Buena Vista Home Entertainment
  VHS/DVD Release Date, March 2002
  Web sites: *www.amazon.com*; *www.babyeinstein.com*; *www.babycenter.com*
  Mozart's music has been shown to affect people of all ages in positive ways. Baby Mozart is a playful, imaginative introduction for infants and toddlers to the music of Mozart. Little eyes will light up at the images of brightly colored toys and visually captivating objects, while little ears will love the carefully arranged music and amusing sound effects.
- Baby MacDonald: A Day on the Farm
  Studio: Walt Disney Home Video
  DVD Release Date, March 2004
  Web sites: *www.amazon.com*; *www.babyeinstein.com*
  This DVD is a fun-filled introduction to the sights and sounds of a farm. It features live-action images and engaging visuals of puppets, children, toys, and real-world objects. It combines traditional nursery rhymes with the beautiful music of Schubert, Schumann, and Strauss.
- Baby Noah Animal Expedition DVD
  Studio: Buena Vista Home Entertainment
  DVD Release Date, October 2004
  Web sites: *www.amazon.com*; *www.babyeinstein.com*
  This is a musical introduction to animals around the globe. It features animals from the rainforest, the outback, and more, and includes the music of Beethoven, Mozart, and Strauss.

○ Childproofing and Safety
  Keeping our children safe is a prime concern for all parents. We want to do everything we can to protect our children from harm or injury. The following videos will show you how to childproof your home and what to do in case of illness or accidents by teaching you first-aid techniques and CPR. Knowing what to do in an emergency situation could save your child's life. Every parent, grandparent, and childcare giver should take an infant CPR and first-aid

class. Have one of these videos on hand to review often so the techniques will remain fresh in your mind.

- Baby and Child CPR
  Studio: Consumervision
  VHS Release Date, June 2001
  Web site: *www.amazon.com*
  Parents of young children eager to learn the basics of cardiopulmonary resuscitation (CPR) and choking relief will welcome this straightforward instructional video. Based on recent guidelines for pediatric CPR set by the American Heart Association, the program offers separate sections on administering to infants (children under one year old) and kids ages one to eight. A winner of Parent's Choice and Kids First awards, the video offers clear, step-by-step instructions accompanied by demonstrations of proper lifesaving techniques.

- Infant Emergencies and CPR . . . When You Least Expect It
  VHS Release Date, June 2000
  Web site: *www.amazon.com*
  This video offers anyone who is responsible for the care of an infant the opportunity to learn primary prevention strategies and emergency-response techniques specific to infancy.

- The Babyproof Home Video
  Web site: *www.safetycareinc.com*
  Endorsed by the American Academy of Pediatrics, this video takes you on an informative room-by-room safety tour that includes the kitchen, bathroom, nursery, and other areas of the home. Locate home hazards and protect your baby from harm using the information in this program.

- The CPR Review for Infants and Children
  Studio: North Star Entertainment, LLC
  VHS Release Date, June 1999
  Web site: *www.amazon.com*
  A must to own if you have children. If something happens, you will know just how to administer CPR quickly and effectively.

Chapter 29
Music Library

○ Prenatal Music
Research findings support the theory that listening to classical music is good for you and your unborn baby. Studies show that your baby listens actively from about the sixth month on. It is believed that playing music for your baby in utero enhances early brain development; promotes creativity, language, and reasoning; and strengthens concentration and memory.

- Mozart for Mothers-to-Be
  Label: Philips
  CD Release Date, April 1996
  Web sites: *www.amazon.com*; *www.bn.com*
  This heartwarming collection of Mozart "lullabies" creates a loving atmosphere that will be a source of inspiration to you during this special time. Mozart's enchanting music will soothe, relax, and entertain both you and your child for years to come.

- Pregnancy Relaxation: A Guide to Peaceful Beginnings By Dana Schardt
  CD Release Date, March 2000
  Web site: *www.amazon.com*
  This CD enables you to blend mind/body/spirit, eases discomforts in pregnancy, enhances sleep, reduces anxiety and stress, assists in preparation for labor and delivery, and allows you to spend special time with your baby-to-be.

- Ultrasound: Music for the Unborn Child
  Label: RCA
  CD Release Date, April 1999
  Web sites: *www.amazon.com*; *www.bn.com*
  This is a great CD for Mom and baby. Listen to the music of Mozart, Vivaldi, Debussy, Chopin, and Bach, and let this

selection of soothing sounds and gentle rhythms serenade you and your baby. This beautiful CD is sure to be a favorite for many years to come.

I found this CD relaxing during pregnancy and we use it just as often in the nursery.—Monica

○ Classical Music for Babies
Studies have shown that babies who listen to classical music show increased verbal ability, spatial recognition, intelligence, comprehension, memory, and intuition.

- Baby Bach
  Label: Buena Vista Entertainment
  Web site: *www.babyeinstein.com*
  Johann Sebastian Bach's music stimulates your baby and helps him become familiar with instrumental sounds.

- Baby Beethoven by Baby Einstein
  Web site: *www.babyeinstein.com*
  Your baby is introduced to Beethoven's works with the sounds of flutes and xylophones. Selections include "Minuet in G," "Rondo in C," "Pathetique," and "Für Elise."

- Baby Mozart by Buena Vista Entertainment
  Web site: *www.babyeinstein.com*
  Mozart's classical music will calm and soothe your baby. It will help your baby relax and fall asleep easily.

○ Bedtime Lullabies
There's nothing more soothing than falling asleep to the soft, gentle sounds of a sweet lullaby. These CDs are sure to lull your baby to sleep.

● Lullaby Themes for Sleepy Dreams by Rock Me Baby
Web site: *www.babycenter.com*
Winner of the Parent's Choice Gold Award, *Lullaby Themes for Sleepy Dreams* will help your baby fall asleep with Susie Tallman's soothing vocals and acoustic guitar. *Lullaby Themes for Sleepy Dreams* features eighteen lilting versions of some of the world's best-known lullabies.

● Lullaby Classics by Baby Einstein
Web sites: *www.babyeinstein.com*; *www.babycenter.com*
This is a peaceful musical collection to soothe and calm little ones to sleep. It includes Brahms's "Lullaby" and other relaxing and delightful selections.

● Night Night Time by Sleep Lullabies
Web site: *www.sleeplullabies.com*
Nine soothing lullabies set to the calming rhythm of a mother's heartbeat to help crying children and fussy babies relax and fall into a safe, peaceful sleep.

○ White Noise CDs for Relaxing Baby
Babies find the gentle sounds of white noise very calming. White noise can soothe colicky babies and help them relax and fall gently to sleep.

● Baby's Blow Dryer CD
Web site: *www.sleeplullabies.com*
Your fussy baby will quiet down to the amazingly comforting sound of a running blow dryer mixed with white noise.

● Baby's Electric Fan CD
Web site: *www.sleeplullabies.com*
The steady, comforting hum of an electric fan can gently lull baby to sleep.

● Baby's First White Noise CD
Web site: *www.sleeplullabies.com*
This CD consists of one full hour of 100 percent pure white noise to soothe and calm your baby.

● Baby's Vacuum Cleaner CD
Web site: *www.sleeplullabies.com*
Parents swear that the comforting combination of vacuum cleaner sounds mixed with white noise helps their baby go to sleep.

Appendix
Online Shopping for Baby

With the hectic lifestyles so many of us lead today, shopping online has become a real convenience. If you are busy working, have other children to take care of, are on bed rest because of a high-risk pregnancy, or just don't have a lot of time to shop, the following Web sites, listed in alphabetical order, will make shopping a breeze. Listed are some general Web sites where you will find most or all of the products you'll need for your baby. Some Web sites that specialize in certain items are also listed.

GENERAL WEB SITES

www.ababy.com
www.ababyoutlets.com
www.albeebaby.com
www.amazon.com
www.aventamerica.com
www.babiesrus.com
www.babyage.com
www.babyant.com
www.babybazaar.com
www.babybungalow.com
www.babycatalog.com
www.babycenter.com
www.babydelight.com
www.babydepot.com
www.babynet.com
www.babyproofingplus.com
www.babystyle.com
www.babysupermall.com
www.babysupermarket.com
www.babyultimate.com
www.babyuniverse.com
www.baby-wise.com
www.babywizards.com
www.badgerbasket.com

www.barebabies.com
www.bcfdirect.com
www.bestbabygear.com
www.bestbuybaby.com
www.buybuybaby.com
www.comfortfirst.com
www.cyberbabymall.com
www.dreamtimebaby.com
www.ebabysuperstore.com
www.etoys.com
www.fisher-price.com
www.jcpenny.com
www.kidstockmontana.com
www.kidsurplus.com
www.lullabylane.com
www.macys.com
www.mailorderexpress.com
www.mastermindtoys.com
www.mommyshop.com
www.mybirthcare.com
www.naturalbabycareproducts.com
www.netkidswear.com
www.ninemonths-etc.com
www.onestepahead.com

www.sassybaby.com
www.sears.com
www.showeryourbaby.com
www.smartstartbaby.com
www.target.com

www.thebabyoutlet.com
www.therightstart.com
www.travelingtikes.com
www.walmart.com

MANUFACTURER WEB SITES

www.babybuddy.com
www.babyeinstein.com
www.babygap.com
www.babytrend.com
www.badgerbasket.com
www.basiccomfort.com
www.bonnybabies.com
www.boppy.com
www.britaxusa.com
www.coscojuvenile.com
www.dexproducts.com
www.evenflo.com
www.fisher-price.com
www.gerber.com
www.gerberchildrenswear.com
www.gracobaby.com
www.infantino.com
www.jlchildress.com
www.jmason.com
www.johnsonsbaby.com

www.kidco.com
www.kiddopotamus.com
www.kolcraft.com
www.kushies.com
www.leachco.com
www.learningcurve.com
www.manhattanbaby.com
www.medela.com
www.munchkininc.com
www.mustela.com
www.pacifeeder.com
www.perego.com
www.playtexbaby.com
www.podee.com
www.princelionheart.com
www.safety1st.com
www.sassybaby.com
www.thefirstyears.com
www.tinylove.com

WEB SITES THAT SPECIALIZE

Baby Bedding

If you're looking for a special nursery theme or just some really cute
bedding, the following Web sites are
good places to start. You will also
find these brands on some of the
general Web sites.
www.babybeddingtown.com
www.babydreams.com
www.babymartex.com
www.cottontaledesigns.com
www.glennajean.com
www.hoohobbers.com

www.kidsline.com
www.lambsandivy.com
www.patchkraft.com

Breastfeeding Mothers

www.aventamerica.com
www.breastfeed-essentials.com
www.lansinoh.com
www.medela.com
www.mybreastpump.com
www.pumpinpal.com
www.whisperwear.com

Childproofing Equipment

www.childsafety.com
www.kidco.com
www.perfectlysafe.com
www.safeandsecurebaby.com
www.safebeginnings.com
www.safe-tots.com
www.totsafe.com

Cloth Diapers

Many expectant moms want to use cloth diapers instead of disposable diapers. The following Web sites have a wide variety of cloth diapers, diaper wraps, and diaper covers.

www.babycottonbottoms.com
www.bummies.com
www.clothdiaper.com
www.diapersite.com
www.kellyscloset.com
www.thebabymarketplace.com
www.tinytush.com

Colicky-Baby Products

Colicky babies can drive parents up the wall. The following Web sites specialize in products to help calm and soothe colicky babies.

www.colicshop.com
www.crybabyshop.com

Drugstores

If you're looking for particular medications, baby bath products, or other baby-care necessities, these Web sites should have them.

www.americarx.com
www.drugstore.com
www.familymeds.com
www.longs.com
www.medshopexpress.com
www.riteaid.com
www.walgreens.com

Nursery Furniture

If you're looking to buy nursery furniture by the piece or as a complete room group, the following Web sites have beautiful furniture in many different styles and wood finishes.

www.angelline.com
www.armsreach.com
www.childcraftind.com
www.dutailier.com
www.milliondollarbaby.com
www.rumbletuff.com
www.simmonsjp.com
www.storkcraft.com
www.thenewparentsguide.com

Preemie-Baby Products

It can often be hard to find diapers, clothing, and other necessities for premature or small babies. The following Web sites specialize in products for preemies.

www.babiesadvantage.com
www.childmed.com
www.nurtureplace.com
www.preemie.com

Strollers

The following Web sites specialize in strollers and stroller accessories.

www.arunningstroller.com
www.babyjogger.com
www.babystrollershop.com
www.bobstrollers.com
www.combistrollers.com
www.inglesina.com
www.kelty.com
www.maclarenbaby.com
www.mountainbuggy.com
www.strollandgo.com
www.strollers.com
www.strollercenter.com
www.strollerdepot.com

Index

Enemas, 4
Entertaining toys, 257–58
Episiotomy, 12
Exercise equipment. *See* Activity equipment
Exersaucers, 184–86

Feeding, 170–83, **267–68**. *See also* Bottles and nipples; Breastfeeding
accessories (utensils, etc.), 181–83, 234–37
baby-food processors, 182–83
formula feeding options, 14
powdered formula, 180–81
reference resources, 290–91
schedule, 90–91
traveling accessories, 234–37
Fever reducer, 37, 152
Fireplace safety, 82
Fire safety, 83
First-aid, 36–41, 298–99, 310–11
Fitness books, 282–85, 291, 304–7
Formula. *See* Bottles and nipples; Feeding
Furniture, **262–63**. *See also* Bassinets; Changing table; Cradles; Crib(s)
co-sleepers/accessories, 118–19
dressers, 115, 116–17
glider rocker, 117
highchairs and booster seats, 192–97, 232, **269**
ottoman, 117–18
safety tips and products, 64–67

Gas-relief drops, 152
Gates, safety, 77–80
Glycerin suppositories, 152
Grooming products, 146–48. *See also* Bath-time essentials
Growth charts, 138

Handprint sets, 140
Hangers, 127
Health and safety information, 86–89, 298–99. *See also* Childproofing home; Emergency phone numbers
Health-care products, 150–53, **265–66**. *See also* Skin-care products

Highchairs and booster seats, 192–97, 232, **269**
Highchair toys, 251–52, 258
Hospital, 2–7. *See also* Packing for hospital
arriving at, in labor, 7
choosing, factors to consider, 2–3
familiarizing yourself with, 3–6
preregistration, 6–7
questions to ask, 4–7
Hot and cool gel packs, 235–36
Humidifiers, 153

Jumpers, 186–87

Keepsakes, 140–41, **264–65**, 300–301
Kitchen safety, 71–73
Knobs and pulls, 139

Labor, induction/augmentation, 11
Labor, plan for, 10–11, 12
Lamps, 126
Lap pads, 103
Laundry products, 134–35
Layette, 94, 99–104
Lead testers, 83
Lotions/skin-care, 154–57

Massage, baby, 308–9
Master shopping lists, **260–73**
baby gear, **268–72**
bath-time essentials, **265**
feeding time, **267–68**
health-care products, **265–66**
keepsakes, **264–65**
newborn necessities, **260–62**
nursery accessories, **264**
nursery furniture, **262–63**
nursery necessities, **263**
nursery niceties, **263–64**
products for nursing mothers, **266–67**
skin-care products, **266**
toys, **272–73**
traveling accessories, **272**
Mattresses. *See* Bedding
Medicine
anesthesia/pain medication, 11–12

About the Author

ELAINE FARBER has made a career of loving and nurturing babies in a variety of environments. She has worked in hospital nurseries, run a daycare center, provided consultation to expectant parents, and served as nanny for families with newborns, 90 percent of whom were twins, triplets, or quadruplets. Elaine's love for children has prompted her to investigate and review a multitude of products in real-world conditions. She knows firsthand which items are the easiest to use and the safest for baby.

Elaine has coached families through every aspect of early parenting, from selecting the right hospital to choosing the proper diapers. Many families in the San Francisco Bay Area revere and trust her, and she is known throughout the multiples community for her remarkable ability to care for twins, triplets, and quadruplets with ease.

In addition to raising three children of her own, Elaine has been a child-care professional for more than twenty-five years. Her hands-on experience, combined with her knowledge of today's trends as well as timeless solutions, make her the ideal author for this book, with a voice that parents everywhere can trust.